Praise for *Confronting Your Spouse's Porr*

"Whereas other books on pornography addic
and individual, this book recognizes that o
combating addiction is support and accounta
other. Praise to spouses willing to confront and be confronted."

Rick Schatz, President & CEO
National Coalition for the Protection of Children & Families

"If you want to confront a spouse or finally disclose secrets about problematic sexual behaviors, this book provides excellent advice. Combining both research and clinical experience Reid and Gray offer practical suggestions to help couples honor their values, get through the turmoil, and heal from this challenging situation."

M. Deborah Corley, Ph.D.
Author of Disclosing Secrets *and* Embracing Recovery,
Clinical Supervisor of Sante Center for Healing, Argyle, Texas

"Looking back, I wish this book had been available during my 25 year addiction to pornography. I am now free from the grip of my addiction and have devoted my life to combating its rampant effects. Rory Reid and Dan Gray have acknowledged one of the most powerful influences to catalyze change—a devoted spouse or partner. With partners and spouses working together, real change will come about."

Phil Burress, President, Citizens for Community Values,
Public policy organization officially associated with Focus on the Family

"This book sheds light on an aspect of sexual behavior and addiction that is all too common in this age of Internet use. The authors have articulated a concise and relevant model that provides readers with the tools necessary to begin healing the shame, loneliness, and helplessness that often accompanies this extreme retreat from intimacy."

Sheila Garos, Ph.D.
Assistant Professor of Psychology, Texas Tech University

"Wives whose husbands are hooked on pornography contact Morality in Media on a regular basis. They describe men who broke their hearts, who lost interest in them sexually or forced sex on them, who committed adultery, who pose a risk to their children. They want to know what they should do; most want to help their husbands. This readable, no-nonsense book provides common sense and professional counsel for both the injured spouse and the addicted spouse."

Robert Peters,
President, Morality in Media

"Since the advent of the Internet, pornography consumption has been eroding relationships at an unprecedented rate. This book represents the work of two therapists who have treated hundreds of affected couples and provides invaluable insight into how to overcome pornography's influence and cultivate healthier marital intimacy. A wide range of topics are handled with a delicate sensitivity to the intense range of feelings this kind of issue evokes, while at the same time offering practical, concrete solutions."

Jill C. Manning, Ph.D.
Marriage and Family Therapist

"With great sensitivity, Rory Reid and Dan Gray address what is perhaps the fastest growing serious problem in married life—addiction to pornography. This book shows how important honesty, trust and caring are to a marriage, and how they can strengthen and even save a family."

Most Reverend George Niederauer, Ph.D.,
Archbishop of San Francisco

"*Confronting Your Spouse's Pornography Problem* is a highly instructive and timely resource for helping couples restore trust and earn forgiveness when a partner is addicted to pornography."

Janis Abrahms Spring, Ph.D.
Author of How Can I Forgive You? *and* After the Affair

CONFRONTING YOUR SPOUSE'S PORNOGRAPHY PROBLEM

Rory C. Reid, LCSW
Dan Gray, LCSW

SILVERLEAF
PRESS

Silverleaf Press Books are available exclusively
through Independent Publishers Group.

For details write or telephone
Independent Publishers Group, 814 North Franklin St.
Chicago, IL 60610, (312) 337-0747

Silverleaf Press
8160 South Highland Drive
Sandy, Utah 84093

Table of Contents

Introduction

An increasing number of people are turning to the Internet for pornography and related activities such as illicit chat rooms, cybersex, solicitation of prostitutes, or worse, predatory behavior towards minors. In most cases, secrecy enables and perpetuates these problems, which have devastating effects on marriages. Unfortunately, most people do not know how to appropriately confront a spouse who may be indulging in these behaviors.

It is common for these spouses to report, "I knew what was going on but remained silent because I didn't know what to say," or "I really didn't want to face the pain of confronting him, so I avoided the issue and even denied it was happening." These individuals claim that remaining silent reduces the potential for conflict. Some worry that confronting a spouse about their use of pornography may jeopardize the marriage. They choose to ignore the "elephant standing in the middle of the room" despite their own feelings of disappointment, hurt, or frustration, and instead tiptoe around it, pretending it doesn't exist or affect how they think or feel. Some discover a problem and immediately confront their spouses with inappropriate comments or actions that may unintentionally make the problem worse.

Ironically, many spouses who participate in these unhealthy activities desire to abandon their behavior and free themselves from a double life but do not know how to disclose their secrets to their partner. They see disclosure as a frightening experience. They fear the adverse reactions or consequences they may encounter.

A typical comment is, "If I told my spouse, she would leave me." Although such a reaction is possible, the majority of spouses remain in the marriage. Some pornography users defiantly indulge themselves despite the disapproval of their spouses and other possible consequences. If healthy intimacy is a marital goal, pornography problems must be confronted and discussed.

Honest disclosure is a necessary step in dissolving the secrecy that fuels pornography addiction and in establishing a relationship built on trust. This openness will include awareness and acceptance of awkward or uncomfortable truths. Unfortunately, many want to avoid talking about such things because it's too painful. Although discussing sensitive issues may be difficult, it is a necessary part of achieving a healthier relationship.

This book contains suggestions and advice the authors have found helpful in counseling (1) those who have confronted their spouses regarding the use of pornography and related behaviors, and (2) those who have disclosed to their spouses problems with compulsive sexual behavior and who are anxious to begin the process of healing. It contains principles that have proven effective in setting couples on the path to overcoming the influence of pornography on individuals, marriages, and families.

The Structure of the Book

This book is divided into four sections. The first section contains information for a spouse who fears his or her partner may be struggling with the effects of compulsive pornography use. It discusses the potential impact such behavior can have on marriages, and models strategies successfully used by others to verify and confront the problem in a constructive way.

The second section of the book is written to those who are using pornography. It provides compelling reasons for disclosing the full extent of the problem to a partner. It contemplates issues that compulsive pornography users are likely to confront as they contemplate changing the dynamics of their situation.

The third section of the book answers the question, "what now?" It discusses the role of forgiveness and trust in rebuilding healthy intimacy. It introduces principles and strategies gathered from clinical experience, research, and the testimonies of clients who have overcome harmful patterns together.

The fourth section of the book reexamines the need for both members of the marriage partnership to receive support during the painful process of recovery. The truth of the matter is that when compulsive pornography use impacts a marriage, it is not just one spouse's problem. It takes the commitment and consistent effort of both partners working together to realize change and rescue the relationship.

Disclaimer

Compulsive pornography use is predominantly a male problem, though growing numbers of females also struggle with pornography. For the purpose of simplifying discussions throughout this book, the authors have used the pronoun *he* to refer to a person with a pornography problem and the pronoun *she* to refer to the non-participating spouse although the behaviors, principles and strategies discussed in this book are not gender specific and are equally appropriate to couples where the addicted partner is a woman.

Defining Pornography

The word "pornography" can denote a wide range of materials and sexual behaviors. For the purposes of this book, the words *pornography* and *sexual behaviors* or *related behaviors* are intended to encompass pornography, cybersex, infidelity, predatory behaviors on the Internet or offline, illicit chat room discussions, and so on.

Confidentiality

The stories used in this work reflect experiences in the lives of clients treated by the authors. In every case, details that would identify the clients have been slightly altered to preserve client anonymity and confidentiality.

SECTION 1:
Confronting Pornography Problems

1. Does My Spouse Have a Problem?

In today's world, many spouses are concerned about the availability and accessibility of pornography. The negative and destructive influence of pornography has adversely affected many lives. You may share these same concerns. You may suspect, through actual evidence or an intuitive impression, that your spouse is using pornography. Accurately discerning whether or not a spouse is struggling with pornography is a difficult yet important first step in confronting and coping with your suspicions. The following chapters will assist you in accurately addressing these difficult issues as you assess the problems and develop a game plan to deal with them in a productive, appropriate, and efficient manner.

Determining whether or not your spouse has a pornography problem is a careful balancing act. Some spouses use the excuse of incomplete or insufficient information to dismiss behavior that should be confronted. One woman, despite her frustration and disgust, excused her husband's pornography habit because she inaccurately assumed it was part of normal male behavior. When his habit later led to a cyber affair,[1] she expressed regret about not confronting the behavior sooner. Another woman grew suspicious of her husband's late-night computer activities, which he said were "work related." Rather than expressing her concern, she quietly went to bed each night. A few months later she discovered that her suspicions were accurate and her husband had been viewing pornography. Both of these examples represent situations where more information should have been gathered and behavior should have been confronted.

Signs of an Existing Problem

Suspicions often arise long before inappropriate behavior is discovered in marriages. There are several signs that may indicate a problem with pornography exists. Some of these signs include:

- Loss of interest in sexual relations or insatiable sexual appetite
- Introduction of unusual or bizarre sexual practices in the relationship
- Diminished emotional, physical, social, spiritual, and intellectual intimacy
- Neglect of responsibilities
- Increased isolation (such as late night hours on the computer); withdrawal from family
- Easily irritated, irregular mood swings or depressed mood
- Unexplained absences or financial transactions
- Preference for masturbation over sexual relations with spouse
- Evidence of hiding computer usage
- Unexpected packages in the mail
- Sexual relations that are rigid, rushed, without passion, and detached

If these signs are present in a marriage, there may be a problem. Many women often initially doubted their intuition which ultimately proved accurate. This however, is not always the case. One spouse became extremely agitated when she discovered pornographic images in the temporary Internet files folder on the family computer. She assumed her husband was indulging in pornography and imagined the devastation that the marriage would suffer as a result of his behavior. When he came home from work, she burst into tears and immediately began attacking him. As the details unfolded, the couple discovered that their son's teenage friend was responsible. Even if the friend had not confessed, other explanations could have accounted for the presence of the images. For example, various Internet marketing techniques exist that use new computer technology to send pornographic images to a home computer without anyone's knowledge. Thus, it is always important to gather sufficient information and consider various possibilities before concluding that there is a problem.

What If I Suspect But I'm Not Sure?

If a problem is suspected, you can simply say "I'm concerned that you may be struggling with a pornography problem and would like to talk to you about some of my feelings and thoughts that are unsettling for me." If a spouse adamantly denies a problem but suspicions persist, other routes can help you explore potential concerns. For example, technology is now available to help concerned spouses verify suspicions they may have about computer usage in the home: they can install computer software programs capable of monitoring online activity. Many of these programs can be installed undetected in a "stealth" mode and can gather information such as how often pornography is being accessed, which pornography sites are being explored, and the duration of time being spent accessing the material. These programs can also provide vital information regarding the frequency and severity of the problem. Furthermore, if the participating spouse chooses to deny viewing pornography, the program can produce evidence to the contrary. We recommend installing monitoring software on family computers whether or not a pornography problem is suspected, especially if there are children in the home.

Although problems may begin on the Internet, it is important to realize that the potential exists for escalation into offline activities. Therefore, when a pornography problem is addressed, it may expose other sexual activities. As the receiver of a disclosure, you should be prepared to learn of other related behaviors in addition to the viewing of pornography.

If you suspect but are unsure whether there is a problem, it is appropriate to communicate your concerns to your spouse. Perhaps some of the signs listed above may be part of your concerns. Listen and be prepared to give him the benefit of the doubt. If there really is a problem, time will usually expose any inappropriate behaviors.

What If It's Not Considered Pornography, But I'm Uncomfortable With It?

Each person must determine what constitutes a problem. Where do you draw the line? What if material that has traditionally not been considered pornographic leads to your spouse's objectification of others? If your husband is sexually aroused by the Swimsuit Edition of *Sports Illustrated* or spends time fantasizing about the women in your *Victoria's Secret* magazine, how does this make you feel? Is this appropriate? If you're uncomfortable, there is a problem, regardless of whether the material is generally considered pornographic. If your husband is using material to facilitate fantasies about other women, this is inappropriate. If you are hurt by such behavior, remember that your feelings are valid and need to be expressed.

Harmful Effects of Pornography

Is there room in your relationship for pornographic magazines, movies, or images flickering on a computer screen? Producers of adult content would have you believe that consumption of pornography is a "guy thing" or that it's "just harmless fun." These marketing tactics attempt to normalize such behavior so it is more widely accepted. Other tactics attempt to demean any woman who would object to her husband's pornography habits. One magazine depicted a cartoon that mocked a wife who was frustrated with her husband's pornography magazines. The cartoon implied that the wife's complaints were unjustified and, in fact, presented her to the reader as a nagging, paranoid woman.

Regardless of these marketing strategies, pornography is harmful and has led to numerous problems for married couples. Pornography teaches a fraudulent message about human intimacy. It portrays both men and women as objects with insatiable sexual appetites or with unrealistic physical capabilities. Non-committal sexual relations with multiple partners are normalized in pornographic material while monogamous relationships are viewed as cumbersome and undesirable. Distorted views of perverted sex acts are presented as exciting and acceptable. In some cases, viewers observe unhealthy sexual behavior they may have never considered until it was presented in the salacious material. Aspects of intimacy such as communication and tender affection are omitted from pornography, as are consequences for promiscuous sexual behavior, such as sexually transmitted diseases and unwanted pregnancies. Such is the message that pornography producers would have us believe—that it is "harmless fun." It is not harmless, and if your spouse is turning to pornography instead of working to develop healthy intimacy in your marriage, there is a problem and you have a right to confront it.

Pornography has many devastating effects on marriage relationships. Some of the most common effects are:

- Decreased trust and feelings of betrayal
- Distorted views of sexual intimacy
- Decreased emotional, spiritual, and physical intimacy
- Decreased sensitivity, tenderness, and kindness
- Financial instability, including loss of employment
- Decreased mental and physical health
- Strained communications and increased marital conflict
- Increased risk of divorce

Because pornography impacts so many core dimensions of marriage, both partners must be committed to tackling the effects together if the marriage is to be preserved.

Is It My Fault?

Spouses often wonder if the problem is their fault. One woman reported:

My husband began using porn as a teenager. What was once an adolescent hobby became the "other woman" in our marriage. At first it was our intimacy that suffered. Then, his pastime grew into an addiction which then started to include more serious forms of "adultery." He was going to strip bars and sleeping with prostitutes. He was often late, with poor excuses. I noticed our money disappearing and never suspected he was spending nearly $500 a week to feed his addiction. . . . I felt responsible, ugly, ashamed, alone and hopeless. Why would he look at another woman unless I wasn't pretty or sexy enough? Friends rejected my idea that his porn use was ruining our relationship. They told me to be sexier, more sexually responsive and available so that he wouldn't look elsewhere. I tried all these things only to find they didn't work. I ended up feeling like a failure, as a wife and a lover.[2]

This woman, like many others, came to realize that her husband's behavior had nothing to do with her. She was not responsible for his decision to use pornography. One of the most important truths a spouse can realize is that *his* problem is not *her* fault. There are many reasons why he may choose to develop a pornography habit. These reasons may include

- Attempts to escape unhealthy shame about himself, possibly caused by childhood neglect, deprivation of needs, family dysfunction, or abuse
- A desire to be wanted or validated without investing in a relationship
- A coping mechanism used to deal with stress or as a reward for accomplishments
- Inability or fear of developing healthy intimacy
- Boredom and curiosity
- Escape into a fantasy world that pretends to meet his unmet, unrealistic expectations

Regardless of the reason, this problem would have likely developed whether he was married to you or someone else. It is not your fault, and you do not have to tolerate such behavior. The next several chapters will address how you can appropriately confront these issues.

Notes

1. A cyber affair is one where intimacy is shared with another person over the Internet. These relationships can lead to offline encounters where sexual relations occur.
2. *It's Not Your Fault*, National Coalition Against Pornography Pamphlet. www.nationalcoalition.org

2. Reacting to the Discovery of Pornography

Discovering your partner's use of pornography can be very painful. It is often accompanied by a variety of mixed emotions, thoughts, and reactions. Your feelings may include any or all of the following: anger, betrayal, rejection, confusion, depression, disappointment, fear, guilt, responsibility, frustration, feeling unloved, despair, abandonment, rage, disgust, indifference, denial, helplessness, hopelessness, bitterness, resentment, powerlessness, discouragement, loneliness, uncertainty, doubt, hesitancy, devastation, distrust, worthlessness, suspiciousness, alienation, victimization, humiliation, anguish, and even relief. These feelings are normal and you have every right to feel them if you discover your spouse has a pornography problem.

One of these reactions, denial, is very common. A person might say, "My spouse would never do something like this." Denial can occur if the truth is too difficult to accept. The behavior may be interpreted as, "He doesn't love me," a thought so hurtful that denial becomes the defense mechanism to escape from or avoid the pain. Another characteristic of denial is shock that your "predictable" spouse could be guilty of such conduct. This reaction is understandable because many individuals who turn to pornography are successful and intelligent people. Political leaders, attorneys, business people, and even some religious leaders have sought help for problems related to pornography. These individuals appear so untarnished in public that it would be difficult to imagine them living "double lives." Dr. Victor Cline, psychologist and emeritus professor at the University of Utah, found that some of his most intelligent patients were among the most vulnerable. They appeared to have a greater capacity to fantasize, which heightened the intensity of their sexual experience and were thus more susceptible to being conditioned toward addictions.[1]

In order to compensate for the guilt and shame of his double life, a pornography consumer may excel in other areas. He becomes the best softball coach, church leader, or husband in an attempt to feel good about himself. One father reported that every time he acted out, he would feel so guilty he would come home from work with flowers and chocolates or a new outfit for his wife. He would do the dishes and the laundry and read the children bedtime stories. Much of this behavior was an attempt to reduce the shame he felt.[2] It was understandable that his wife was in complete shock and denial when her husband's pornography habit was uncovered and she was faced with the reality that he wasn't everything she thought he was.

Some individuals eventually end up confessing to their spouses because the burden they carry is too great. Although this confession is admirable and requires courage, it does not diminish responsibility for the behavior. Accountability and acceptance of consequences for inappropriate behavior are essential if healing is to occur. Part of this responsibility includes sensitivity to, and complete tolerance of, the non-offending spouse's expressions of hurt and anguish as the indiscretions are disclosed. An adverse reaction is not only normal but can also be an important part of helping the offending spouse recognize the pain and sorrow that inappropriate actions have caused. This can be an important beginning step toward reconnecting the addict with feelings that have been suppressed or dismissed in order to rationalize indulging in his destructive behavior.

Thoughts and feelings of anger and frustration are common and normal. You are entitled to have these emotions, which can be magnified and even more complicated if you are exposed to drastic consequences such as financial loss or risk of sexually transmitted diseases (if a spouse has engaged in sexual relations outside the marriage). In some cases, the media can become involved if they learn of a story they deem newsworthy. This can further humiliate and embarrass an entire family and is especially damaging.

Some spouses report feeling relief when a discovery occurs. They are grateful to uncover the truth and make sense of behaviors and events for which they suspected inappropriate activities but were never sure. In many cases, the non-participating spouse begins to believe that her thoughts and feelings are distorted—that she is imagining things. Sometimes the offending spouse is so manipulative and deceptive that he convinces the non-participating spouse that she, not he, is the one with the problem. In these situations discovering pornography problems can provide relief in the midst of hurt and pain.

Regardless of what feelings or reactions you may have, such emotions are normal and to be expected. They are a natural reaction to an overwhelming, painful discovery. It is helpful to find a therapist or close friend who can be supportive and validate these thoughts and feelings, letting you know it is permissible to feel those things and reaffirming that you are not to blame.

Furthermore, it is critical for the offending spouse to recognize that he must demonstrate extreme patience and a willingness to accommodate the traumatic feelings his spouse is experiencing. Having created the pain that his spouse and family must suffer, he in turn must be willing to absorb their emotional reactions to the pain he has caused. However, it is also important for the non-offending spouse to recognize that what she does with her feelings is crucial. While appropriately demonstrating emotions is part of honest and open communication, the problem is compounded when a spouse becomes physically, emotionally, verbally, or otherwise abusive toward a husband who has disclosed a sexual problem or pornography habit.

Notes

1. Cline, B. Victor, PhD. *Pornography's Effects on Adults and Children*. New York: Morality in Media, 2001, 3.
2. Understanding the shame dynamic underlying addictive behavior is addressed in Appendix E.

3. Confronting a Spouse

I t is often difficult to know how to react appropriately after discovering a problem. Professional counseling can be helpful in deciding what boundaries to establish and what consequences are appropriate.

It is typical for a spouse to immediately confront her partner after discovering pornography in the home. However, if the confrontation is done while emotions are high, unintended things may be done or said. The offending partner may react to the emotions of his spouse rather than hearing what she is trying to communicate. If you enlist the support of a religious leader or therapist, you will not have to go through this process alone.

Don't Enable

Often a spouse may react to the discovery of her husband's addiction with prolonged silence, which may suggest indifference. Denial and avoidance can also manifest themselves through silence, which then becomes a form of enabling his behavior. Ignoring the problem, whether intentionally or not, is the same as condoning the behavior. Another example of enabling is making excuses to his employer, saying he is ill when in fact he spent the night on the computer viewing pornography. People do this because they are afraid of what might happen if they do confront their spouses.

Don't Accommodate

Making excuses for a spouse also constitutes accommodating the inappropriate behavior. A spouse may think, "It's just a phase" or "He's under a lot of stress." Others report feeling that they are partially to blame. This misperception may inadvertently justify the behavior. Although your spouse may use pornography to cope with stress or other emotional issues, you should not assume responsibility for his choices. Inappropriate behaviors do not need to be tolerated. This is an area where the advice to "choose your battles" is applicable. This is one battle you must choose, and choose to win. Pornography addiction must be fought, not feared.

Establish and Maintain Healthy Boundaries

Sometimes when a spouse is confronted, he may become defensive or attempt to change the focus of the real issue. "How dare you snoop around on my computer!" one man yelled to his wife. This display of anger and outrage is a manipulative tactic. It may be true that inspecting his computer was a violation of privacy. This issue can be discussed at a later time, but for now, the focus is on his behavior, not yours. This man's wife appropriately responded, "We can talk about my snooping later. Right now I want to talk about the pornography."

If behavior becomes abusive or you fear personal harm, leave the house or, if necessary, call the police. If an aversive reaction is anticipated, choose a safe place for the initial confrontation such as the office of a therapist or church leader. You are not on trial and do not need to feel guilty about wanting to extinguish this destructive behavior in your home and marriage.

Maintaining a healthy boundary also means saying no to any sexual requests you may feel are wrong or inappropriate. When individuals consume pornography they are sometimes introduced to bizarre or abnormal forms of human sexuality. In turn, they may attempt to have you act out these inappropriate fantasies. By submitting to these demands for unusual or bizarre sex, the real-life experience powerfully reinforces fantasies fueled by the pornography. This is likely to exacerbate the problem and may increase the likelihood of further requests that are more bizarre or distorted.

Don't Reinforce Distorted Beliefs or Thoughts

People who use pornography to cope with life have numerous distorted thoughts and beliefs (see Appendix D). This creates denial as a means of avoiding pain. It is important to show appropriate empathy for such people. However, reinforcing distorted thoughts and beliefs or showing misplaced sympathy may inadvertently justify the behavior in the offending spouse's mind. For example, the following statement indicates several thinking errors: "You haven't had sex with me for so long I had to have my needs met somehow." This expression is an *excuse* used to *rationalize* sexual behavior beyond the marriage relationship. It also attempts to *redefine* the real problem of the husband's misbehavior by attempting to deflect the *blame* to his spouse. This is emotional *manipulation*. His distorted belief is that with sufficient self-pity and *excuse-making*, his wife will show compassion and excuse the inappropriate behavior. An appropriate response might be, "I'm sorry you feel frustrated about your lack of sex in our marriage, and we should talk about that later. Right now I want to talk about your pornography and masturbation." This response avoids reinforcing any thinking errors while showing respect and validation for the person's feelings about his lack of sex. It also keeps the conversation focused.

Show Understanding without Condoning the Behavior

Understanding a spouse's pornography habit does not imply acceptance or approval of inappropriate behaviors. The following information may help you understand the nature of the problem prior to confronting your spouse. Dr. Patrick Carnes suggests that those who use pornography or sex to deal with problems in life will generally possess some or all of the following distorted core beliefs:

1. *Self Image*: I am basically a bad, unworthy person.
2. *Relationships*: I'm unlovable. People cannot love me as I really am.
3. *Needs*: I can't depend on or trust others to meet my own needs.
4. *Sexuality*: Sex is my most important need.[1]

There are many theories as to how these beliefs develop. Most notable are theories that suggest some lack of attachment or validation during childhood. Children can feel abandoned or abused by their caregivers in numerous ways. Whenever this deprivation occurs there is usually an attempt to try and compensate in order to meet basic human needs. When these children discover pornography and masturbation during their adolescent years, the temporary pleasure of self-stimulation provides an escape from the pain caused by the lack of appropriate nurturing from their primary caregivers. They develop a love/hate relationship with the pornography because it acts as a form of self-medication from inner pain while creating a great sense of shame or guilt from acting out the inappropriate behavior. This shame, which one author[2] refers to as "toxic shame," is compounded with the initial shame they felt about themselves. It is important to understand that this element of shame is common among many compulsive pornography consumers. The difference between a shame-based person and an individual who feels guilt is that a guilt-based person says, "I feel bad about my behavior," whereas a shame-based person says, "I feel bad about who I am" or "Somehow I'm inherently flawed as an individual." Escaping this tremendous sense of shame may be the function of pornography use. The shame-based person turns to pornography—a mere counterfeit for feeling something besides the shame created by the inner pain he feels about himself. (See Appendix E for further discussion of shame and addiction.)

Although this theory may explain why some individuals use pornography and related behaviors as a maladaptive coping behavior in their lives, it does not apply to every situation. Some individuals who have come from healthy families still struggle with these issues. Regardless of the root cause, childhood trauma notwithstanding, those who indulge in sexual improprieties remain responsible for their behavior. Shame and other psychological issues are reasons, not excuses.

Understanding possible explanations for sexually inappropriate behaviors is helpful when confronting a spouse who may be struggling. Many people ask, "Why?" Why would a husband or wife do such a thing? Understanding the concept of toxic shame provides some explanations. Some spouses tend to blame themselves for their husbands' actions with erroneous thoughts such as, "I'm not sexy enough or beautiful enough." An awareness of this shame theory can provide an understanding that it's not about you, it's about your spouse and the unhealthy way he chooses to cope with his problems.

Understanding underlying issues also helps the non-participating spouse to show empathy for her loved one. Realize, however, that expressing empathy and validating his feelings does not mean that you accept, agree with, or approve of his behavior. In fact, while you are showing correct empathy, it is also important to be assertive and clearly communicate your feelings and disapproval of the behavior. For example, after you listen to your spouse discuss his pain, an appropriate response might be, "I'm sorry you feel so much hurt and pain. I can understand how unfair life may seem to you and I want you to know that I love you. But I still feel disappointed and hurt by your behavior and I cannot and will not tolerate it in our home."

Providing support to an offending spouse is a difficult endeavor. It should be done without taking any responsibility for the offensive behavior. Women often take responsibility by thinking they are to blame. This is erroneous, unhealthy thinking. You must understand that the addictive mind is never satisfied. A man with a sexual compulsion could be married to the most attractive woman alive and he would still engage in excessive sexual behavior outside the marriage. The problem is rarely about his spouse.

Communicate Your Feelings, Thoughts, and Concerns

When addressing a spouse, it is important to clearly communicate how you feel and what you expect. This can be done without attacking or shaming. Healthy confrontation is very direct but non-threatening. The focus is on the problem behavior and expressing thoughts and feelings. However, uncontrollable crying, yelling, or screaming may undermine the objectives of the confrontation. The attention will focus too heavily on emotions and the message may be lost. Waiting a few days, or in some cases longer, before confronting the problem may help a spouse reduce the intensity of her emotions. Time may increase objectivity and appropriate responses for both parties. She must take care, however: waiting can become avoidance. Avoidance can create denial and perpetuate secrecy. It is important that the non-offending spouse not let too much time pass.

If you are concerned about your ability to stay in control of your emotions, perhaps you could plan the discussion to take place in the presence of a therapist or religious leader so that interactions can be moderated by a third person.

Notes

1.   Carnes, Patrick, PhD. *Out of the Shadows*. Hazelden Press, Minnesota 1992, 77-81.
2.   Bradshaw, John. *Healing the Shame that Binds You*. Health Communications, Florida 1988.

4. The Discussion: Confronting the Problem

Talking about a pornography problem with a spouse is a difficult task. Maintaining an appropriate communication style can help facilitate this process. There are primarily four styles of communication:

1. Assertive
2. Aggressive
3. Passive
4. Passive-Aggressive

Assertive Communication

In assertive communication, thoughts, desires, and feelings are openly expressed while considering the rights and feelings of others. Reflective listening demonstrates a sincere desire to understand the other person's point of view. Assertive communicators are usually open to negotiation and compromise. When speaking, their voices are relaxed, well modulated, and firm. They maintain good eye contact, and their facial expressions demonstrate interest in the discussion. One spouse effectively expressed to her partner concern over a possible problem with these words: "Honey, I've noticed you've been staying up really late on the computers—sometimes into the early hours of the morning—and I'm feeling really uncomfortable with that. I'm concerned. It makes me nervous." This type of communication allows for an exchange of understanding when sensitive and delicate issues are addressed. Simply stated, assertive communication is an "I count, you count" approach.

Aggressive Communication

Aggressive communication implies, "I count, you don't count." Thoughts and feelings are communicated at the expense of others' rights or interests. Yelling at someone is an example of aggressive communication. Aggressive communication is often laden with sarcasm, contempt, criticism, blaming, name-calling, put-downs, and condemnation. Black-and-white thinking permeates the discussion with statements such as "you always" or "you never." Being right is usually more important than being understood, and listening skills are usually poor. In aggressive communication the issues get lost in emotion.

Passive Communication

Passive communicators avoid being direct as they express feelings, thoughts, or concerns. A passive person will listen to her spouse vent about his problem with pornography and neglect to communicate her anger and frustration with his behavior. This style promotes the idea, "You count, I don't count." Passive communicators usually do not maintain eye contact. Their voices are weak, soft, wavering, and timid. A passive person might say, "I see why you have this problem and I'm sorry I'm making matters worse for you. I should be more understanding. Let's not deal with this now. We can talk about it some other time."

Passive-Aggressive Communication

Passive-aggressive communication says, "I count, you don't count, but I'm not going to tell you that you don't count." It is often non-verbal. For example, one client placed a virus on her husband's computer hoping to damage his files, including all of his pornographic images. She didn't tell him and acted surprised when he complained about having the virus on his computer. Passive-aggressive communication is indirect and usually ineffective.

Effective Communication

When confronting inappropriate behavior, clearly the best communication style is an assertive one. It creates an environment in which both parties can be understood. When a person feels upset and frustrated about a problem, however, maintaining an appropriate communication style can be difficult. Talking about feelings using "I" statements can often help avoid using blaming or judgmental language: "I feel hurt," "I feel upset," "I feel disappointed," "I feel confused." Remember, a feeling is one word. It's easy to begin describing a feeling using "I" and instead communicate a thought using "you." For example, "*I* feel that *you* are inconsiderate" shifts the focus to "you" and constitutes a thought, not a feeling. Be careful to avoid this type of language as it may be misunderstood. Also, identify clearly your true thoughts and feelings before discussing them with your spouse. This approach will help your communication be genuine rather than reactive and will not reflect thoughts that are impulsive and inaccurate.

Effective communication moderates conflict. It does not eliminate it. Many individuals who are uncomfortable with conflict settle for an avoidant or accommodative approach. They may believe that conflict is bad. The reality is that all marriages have some conflict. In fact, if a marriage is void of conflict it is likely that one spouse dominates the other. What makes good marriages great is when couples have learned how to respectively resolve their conflicts. This can be accomplished when both partners use an assertive—"I count, you count"—approach in addressing their differences.

The offending spouse should be sensitive, caring, and willing to listen with an open mind and heart as his wife vents and expresses her hurt and anger. The following example illustrates this point and also reminds us that problems with pornography and related behaviors are not exclusively a male problem. After becoming involved in a cyber affair, one woman confessed to her husband that she felt so alone in their marriage and that he didn't care about her anymore. After listening at some length to her, the husband expressed that he too had felt the distance between them. He told her that he would be willing to address this at a later time, but for the moment, he wanted to address the issue of her online behavior in illicit chat rooms. In this manner, the husband validated the frustration of his wife and agreed to address their marital problems at a later time. As a result, the wife was willing to continue a very sensitive conversation about her own inappropriate behavior. The husband was then able to communicate that her Internet activities were unacceptable and not a solution to their problems.

Even with an assertive approach, discussing a pornography problem can be an extremely daunting task. Nonetheless, it must be confronted if healthy intimacy is to be obtained. If the discussion is done appropriately using effective communication, the difficult task of confronting a spouse will have a greater chance of success.

5. Anticipating Your Spouse's Reaction

After being confronted about inappropriate behaviors, a spouse can react in a variety of ways. Reactions may include denial, anger, blame, guilt, shame, fear, defiance, rage, contrition and remorse, humility, relief, avoidance, withdrawal, humor, sarcasm, or ambivalence. Paying attention to the emotional reactions of your spouse will help you determine how to continue responding to the problem at hand.

Denial

A common reaction is denial. For example, one spouse claimed, "I haven't a clue how those images got on our computer." This may suggest a complete refusal to acknowledge that a problem exists. Another form of denial is minimizing. This form manifests itself when someone admits awareness but minimizes intent. A person may say, "I accidentally came upon a pornography site and that's why those images are on our computer," when in fact, it wasn't an accident at all. Although both responses may at first sound legitimate, if there are many images present or an extensive history of adult web sites in the Internet browser, then the likelihood of it being an accident is remote.

If you have sufficient evidence to suspect or substantiate a serious problem but your spouse denies any inappropriate behavior, then it may be necessary to reaffirm your position more assertively. After listening to her husband adamantly deny any use of pornography, one wife responded, "I've stood at your office door on several occasions when you were staring at pornography on your computer. Each time, it was obvious to me that you were in no hurry to turn your monitor off. I wanted to give you the benefit of the doubt, but realized I could not." This spouse then communicated clearly how she felt about the problem. She also expressed her concern that her husband had attempted to lie in order to keep his behavior a secret. All of this was done in a non-threatening way and her husband confessed to a problem, which they were then able to work through together.

Avoidance and Resistance

Another common reaction to confrontations about pornography use is avoidance and resistance. Avoiding responsibility or accountability for a behavior enables a person to also avoid consequences. One form of avoidance is a dismissive response: "I don't want to talk about it." In this case, denial is replaced with a reluctance to discuss the problem. Another form of avoidance is being constantly unavailable to talk about the problem. "This isn't a good time right now. Talk to me later," replied one spouse. When asked what would be a good time, the response was, "I don't know." This tactic is used to postpone discussing the problem. If it is repeated often enough, some spouses become exhausted and eventually give up trying. An assertive person might respond by saying, "That's not acceptable to me. If you want to postpone this discussion I would appreciate you giving me a time when we can talk about it." When this type of assertiveness is used, a common reaction is anger. It might be helpful to remember that anger is a secondary emotion and that primary emotions causing anger usually include embarrassment, frustration, fear, and guilt. One spouse, recognizing this, told her husband, "I know you're probably afraid to talk about this, but it's important to me. I love you and want to help but can't if you refuse to open up and have a discussion with me." This approach helped her husband feel safe, and he confided in her about his struggles.

Minimizing can also be used to avoid. "I *just* did it *once*," or "It *only* happened a few times." These expressions attempt to make behavior appear insignificant or unimportant. Minimizing often manifests itself with words such as "only," "just," or "once." Information provided is usually vague, unclear, or non-specific so the person listening is incapable of seeing the complete picture and is likely to draw inaccurate conclusions.

Others avoid by redefining the issue, using a tactic commonly known as "changing the subject." One husband told his wife, "I may have looked at a picture or two but it isn't any worse than the romance novels you read or the soap operas you watch." This tactic attempts to take the focus off of his behavior and place it elsewhere. An appropriate response might be, "That might be a valid point that I would be happy to discuss later. Right now I want to talk about the matter of the pornography on the computer."

Another way to redefine the issue is to play the victim. When a person attempts to manipulate a situation through a "poor me" approach, the goal is to avoid responsibility by eliciting pity. If a wife feels sorry for her spouse, she may begin to caretake his emotions at the cost of processing her own. In this manner, the focus is changed and responsibility for behavior is avoided. One husband began to cry, and as he sobbed he began to make excuses for his behavior by blaming it on all the stress he was feeling. His wife began to rescue him by expressing her sorrow for his situation. After the pattern repeated itself several times, she began to resent the fact that she was taken in by his self-pity. This trap could have been avoided had she been more assertive about her feelings from the beginning. This doesn't mean that appropriate empathy and compassion can't be expressed, but it's also important to avoid traps that prevent honest communication of thoughts and feelings.

Defiance

One person became enraged when his spouse confronted him about pornography that was discovered on their computer. The husband responded, "So what. I don't care. It's none of your business. Don't even go near my computer ever again. In fact, I'm going to put a password on it right now because I don't want you touching it!" Defiance, usually manifested through anger, is a symptom of guilt, fear, embarrassment, or frustration.

In most cases, a person who leads a double life works very hard to maintain what is sometimes called "impression management." When all the work of maintaining his good guy image is threatened by exposure of his embarrassing behavior, he may become very angry and defiant. Trying to communicate with someone who demonstrates this behavior will be difficult. It may be more helpful to postpone the discussion until the person is less hostile. An ideal response might be, "I can see this is not a good time to talk with you. We will discuss this later. When would be the best time for you?" If this approach is met with additional defiance, it may be necessary to enlist the help of a therapist to formulate a strategy to address the spouse's resistance. Understanding healthy boundaries, the subject of the next chapter, may provide additional assistance about how to respond to defiance.

Contrition and Remorse

"I'm sorry, I need help, I know it's wrong," responded one person after being confronted by his spouse. It's not uncommon for a spouse to express remorse, request forgiveness, and commit to abandon the behavior. Psychologist Dr. Kimberly Young notes:

> His promises at the time are probably sincere, and most loved ones want to believe the words. A honeymoon period may follow, including intense sexual activity between the couple. Since sex is often regarded as a sign of love, a spouse may be lulled into believing everything is really all right, offer forgiveness, and bind up her wounded spirit and go on. She is later shattered to discover that the unaccounted time and secrecy has returned. If the core issues aren't addressed, relapse is bound to happen.[1]

Understanding the tendency for relapse can help put a contrite or remorseful reaction into perspective. Thus, when someone promises to abandon a problem with pornography, it is best to realize the magnitude of sex addiction problems. Even for those who show remorse, professional assistance is usually required to effectively address compulsive sexual behavior.

If a person appears contrite about his behavior, it is important to be patient in trying to understand him. This neither implies agreement with the behavior nor dismissal of personal feelings. It does suggest receptivity to the offending spouse's feelings and perspective. Most people want to abandon their unhealthy habits because of the tremendous guilt and shame they feel.

Deception

Some individuals will admit wrongdoing and promise to abandon the behavior even though they have no intention of doing so. The confrontation communicates to them that they need to take greater precautions to cover up their behavior. As a result, they agree to change but secretly plan to become more deceptive instead. The difference between this type of person and a person who is contrite and apologetic but relapses to the behavior is that a contrite person actually intends to keep his commitment while a deceptive person does not. Furthermore, if a contrite person has a relapse, he is more likely to disclose additional slips. This demonstrates his desire to break the cycle of secrecy, something a deceptive person is not interested in doing.

Ambivalence

Ambivalence is often at the heart of impulse control disorders associated with pornography. It is a love-hate relationship between the addict and his sexual compulsion. The love comes from the temporary relief he finds using sexual material to facilitate arousal, which becomes a form of self-medication (see Appendix A). However, he feels shame and guilt afterwards and thus develops a hate for the pornography. These coexisting, conflicting feelings create the dilemma about change and represent the core of the ambivalence.

Assessing the Reaction

Regardless of which reaction he demonstrates, it is important that your spouse take responsibility for his own behavior. Letting a loved one have his own responsibility can be difficult. Some try to rescue the spouse, yet experience has shown that this can exacerbate problems rather than help.

Allowing your spouse to take responsibility does not, however, mean leaving him to struggle alone. In fact, even a person who truly desires to change will not likely be successful on his own if he has already experienced several unsuccessful attempts at extinguishing the behavior. Such people tend to do better in a structured environment with a therapist and a support group.

Ultimately a struggling spouse can be influenced, but he is the one who must decide which path he will follow. What he cannot choose are the consequences that accompany his choices. Establishing what boundaries you will have is part of the process that applies consequences for his inappropriate and harmful choices and is the subject of the next chapter.

Notes

1. Young, Kimberly, PhD. *Tangled in the Web*, 83. www.netaddiction.com

6. Establishing Healthy Boundaries

Because it is difficult to help a spouse change his behavior unless he wants to change, the focus of the non-participating spouse should be the development of her own healthy boundaries and sense of self-worth.

Numerous books have been written to address the issues of boundaries and codependency. The purpose of this chapter is to introduce these concepts rather than produce an extensive analysis of what these concepts mean or how to treat them. A list of suggested materials for further reading is found at the end of the chapter.

What are Boundaries?

A boundary is what distinguishes us as separate from others. Much like a fence around a home, it protects us from the outside while giving us an area in which we can feel safe. Each individual is our own gatekeeper and determines who will be allowed to enter the solemn and sacred aspects of our lives.

Pia Mellody, in her work *Facing Codependence*, suggests that boundaries serve three primary functions. First, they prevent others from intruding into our personal space or abusing us. Second, they keep us from intruding into the personal space of others and abusing them. And third, they create a framework or structure that provides us with self-identity, which defines us as individuals.[1]

Anne Katherine defines the function of boundaries in the following manner:

> Boundaries bring order to our lives. As we learn to strengthen our boundaries, we gain a clearer sense of ourselves and our relationship

to others. Boundaries empower us to determine how we'll be treated by others. With good boundaries, we can have the wonderful assurance that comes from knowing we can and will protect ourselves from the ignorance, meanness, or thoughtlessness of others.[2]

There are a number of different boundaries developed throughout our lives. They include emotional, intellectual, physical (including sexual), social-relational, and spiritual boundaries. For example, notice what happens the next time you get into an elevator with a stranger. Do you stand next to the person? Strangers usually stand on opposite sides of the elevator. This is a physical boundary. Is it flexible? What if more people entered the elevator? Most likely the rules for defining your boundary would change and you would be willing to stand closer to a stranger. So it is with all our boundaries. We have rules or beliefs about how we define ourselves in relation to others. These rules affect how we respond to situations and how we interact with others. Although various circumstances may alter our boundaries, each of us determines what the ultimate limits to our boundaries will be.

In marriage relationships, boundaries establish limits that provide the optimum environment for healthy intimacy to flourish. The boundaries for a spouse are usually more transparent than for any other person. *Transparency* represents how well you can see beyond the walls others establish to protect themselves and how well they can see beyond your walls. Transparent people allow others to see their authentic selves. This transparency can enable spouses to know each other more intimately than individuals outside the marriage relationship. It also creates vulnerability to being hurt should a spouse take advantage of the trust that is granted in the context of this unique bond. A boundary violation exists when a person crosses a line that defines our limits. When a spouse indulges in pornography by seeking sexual gratification outside the marriage relationship, a boundary is violated. Trust is broken. Respect is diminished. In response to these violations, boundaries need to be reevaluated and then reaffirmed or redefined. Affirmation of boundary violations may be as simple as communicating the intrusion assertively with the offender. If the offender has intruded unintentionally, he may apologize and take precaution to avoid further violations.

An example of a boundary regarding computer use might be a rule that requires family members to report any accidental exposures to pornography while on the computer. If a spouse has been exposed and informs his partner, the experience can be processed and strategies to avoid additional exposure can be established. It then becomes a learning experience for the family. This boundary also removes shame or guilt that may otherwise be felt because of mistakes or accidents that were unintended. A good boundary is thus established that eliminates secrets and creates an atmosphere of trust in the home regarding computer use.

If a person is selfish, he may not care that he has violated your boundary. In this case, boundaries need to be enforced or reevaluated. The process of reevaluating boundaries may change the relationship's previously defined rules. For example, after one spouse discovered her husband had been masturbating to pornography for an extensive period of time, she redefined her physical boundary and chose not to share sexual intimacy with him until he sought professional help. Such a boundary under regular circumstances would be considered unhealthy because the marriage relationship implies oneness with a spouse that includes sexual intimacy. However, when the trust that enables this closeness to exist is jeopardized by boundary violations, limits can and should be reconsidered.

In one sense, the creation or redefinition of boundaries may seem like implementing consequences. Although this may be true, this is the not the purpose of boundaries. Instead, proper boundaries increase the possibility of having healthy intimacy. Establishing boundaries is an act of love. The message of boundaries is that you care enough about the other person to avoid enabling his harmful behavior in any way. You are communicating that you will not permit him to live beneath himself. Your boundary says "I want to help you be your best self and surely you can't feel good about acting this way." They further communicate that you care enough about yourself that you will not allow others to intentionally hurt you. Boundaries also help prevent you from violating the limits that others have established for themselves.

If a relationship damaged by pornography problems is to be repaired, healthy boundaries must exist before trust and respect can be restored. One woman observed, "If I continued to allow my husband to hurt me in the name of 'compassion' or being 'understanding' I would have become drained until eventually I would resent him and be unwilling to resolve our marriage problems."

Another couple had a disturbing dialogue after the wife attempted to establish healthy boundaries regarding the placement of the computer in the home. Her husband angrily responded, "I don't give a ---- what you think, you better leave my ------- computer alone." She responded, "I feel disrespected when my opinions are dismissed and I will not tolerate profanity and language intended to demean my character. If you continue, I will leave."

Although this woman had no control over her husband's behavior, she had total control over how she chose to react to this situation. Asserting her boundary represented a healthy decision to end being a victim of abusive behavior. Later, when her husband realized she was serious about her boundary, he apologized and expressed a willingness to address her concerns. In this way, the boundary helped her avoid being a victim and helped him develop respect both for her and for himself.

Establishing a Boundary

Women often report they feel trapped or helpless to do anything about their husband's choices. When a woman feels she has no options, this is a clear sign that boundaries need to be established. The first part of establishing a boundary is to identify what makes you feel uncomfortable. The inverse of what is causing the discomfort is where you begin to draw the lines of your boundaries. For example, one woman reported that she felt uncomfortable not having filters on the home computers. In this case, the boundary she would seek to establish is having filters installed on the computers. Another woman established a boundary about deception in the marriage. She told her husband "One mistake doesn't have to become two"—referring to his lying about incidents where he looked at pornography. This was unacceptable to her. In a discussion with her husband she indicated that she would be willing to be patient as he worked on his pornography problem but if he slipped and acted out she would not tolerate him trying to hide his relapses. Her boundary about dishonesty regarding slips helped her husband break the secrecy that enabled him to maintain his behavior.

Codependency

Establishing or enforcing boundaries, as in the previous example, requires assertiveness. Unfortunately, when people have poor boundaries they usually lack assertiveness. Additionally, people with poor boundaries often manifest codependent traits.

Codependency is a term used by the therapeutic community to describe people who maintain a deep-rooted belief that the road to belonging, intimacy, success, acceptance, and validation is dependent upon their ability to please others. As a result of this belief, codependent people become centered externally and their inner self is surrendered in a way where they are manipulated and governed by the thoughts, feelings, and actions of others. Loss of connection with the authentic self is replaced by an obsession to please or control others.

The development of codependency is an extremely complex issue. One explanation suggests that children who suffer some form of neglect or deprivation of their needs develop a low sense of self-worth, which opens the door to numerous dysfunctional attempts by the child to meet those needs. The child's needs are not met in a healthy way, and the child internalizes this experience believing that somehow he or she is flawed.

One author describes how codependency may be developed, defining it as:

> An emotional, psychological, and behavioral condition that develops as a result of an individual's prolonged exposure to, and practice of, a set of oppressive rules—rules which prevent the open expression of feeling as well as the direct discussion of personal and interpersonal problems.[3]

In these situations, codependent traits are developed to compensate for inner pain created by the neglect.

Although these explanations do not fit every situation, they provide insight into some of the common denominators among many codependents. The list of behaviors a codependent person may develop are extensive and may include the following:

1. An impaired ability to differentiate feelings of self and others, which creates a tendency to feel responsible for the feelings of others. You attempt to caretake the emotions of other people.

2. Validation of self depends on the approval, attention, and admiration of others.

3. Feelings of guilt or responsibility when others express strong negative emotions.

4. Service to others is laden with expectations that those you serve will somehow love you or respect you more because of your efforts.

5. Service to others is often at the expense of meeting your own needs.

6. You blame yourself when things go wrong or you feel that you are never good enough.

7. You have great advice for others but don't follow it yourself.

8. A perfectionist tendency where flawless performance defines your value or self-worth.

9. Constant fear of being rejected or abandoned by others.

10. You avoid making demands on others or expressing your true feelings for fear that others may disapprove.

11. You lack assertiveness in sticking up for yourself because you are unsure about what you want or whether it's okay.

12. Presentation of a fake self because you believe others won't accept the authentic you.

13. You feel controlled because of what others think or feel about you.

14. Difficulty sharing or expressing your inner feelings. Most of your relationships lack meaningful intimacy.

15. Black and white thinking—everything is all good or all bad.

16. You are unhappy inside but you pretend everything is okay.

17. Rigid rules define your behavior and you are unforgiving of your own mistakes.
18. Engagement in many activities to feel good about yourself. Often you overextend yourself. You starve for positive comments made about you by others.
19. High expectations that things be done a certain way in order to be acceptable.
20. You feel unappreciated, taken advantage of, or manipulated by others.

If you discover that you possess many of these traits, it is possible that you are struggling with codependency. This does not mean that you are responsible for your spouse's pornography problem. It does suggest that you will cope more effectively with his issues if you first address and resolve your codependency. This can be difficult to accept after all the pain you've suffered living with a spouse who indulges in pornography.

Many individuals are upset when they bring their spouses to therapy to be "fixed" and are told they too can work on becoming healthier people by addressing their codependent behaviors. Although this isn't true for every person, experience suggests that a high percentage of individuals married to someone with unhealthy compulsive behaviors demonstrate at least some codependent tendencies. If this is not addressed concurrently with the offending spouse's issues, it is possible that the offender will begin to develop healthy habits and his spouse will continue to struggle with codependent traits. Furthermore, since one of the traits of a codependent person is a lack of appropriate boundaries, addressing the codependency will also be a necessary part of developing and understanding healthy boundaries.

Beverly Engel provides the following profound insight about the dilemma of codependency:

> The irony is that as much as a codependent feels responsibility for others and takes care of others, she believes deep down that other people are responsible for her. She blames others for her unhappiness and problems, and feels that it's other people's fault that she's unhappy.
>
> Another irony is that while she feels controlled by people and

events, she herself is overly controlling. She is afraid of allowing other people to be who they are and of allowing events to happen naturally. An expert in knowing best how things should turn out and how people should behave, the codependent person tries to control others through threats, coercion, advice giving, helplessness, guilt, manipulation, or domination.[4]

Conclusion

Confronting a spouse who indulges in pornography is a difficult task in any situation. If the spouse is receptive to discussing the problem, couples should work together to develop healthier intimacy and better communication. If your spouse isn't responsive to your confrontation, you will need to decide how you will react to his lack of concern for things that are important to you. As you work through these difficult and complex issues, seek counsel and support from a therapist or church leader. If a spouse is willing to work on the problems, remember to avoid the mentality of our soap opera society that solves complex problems in one or two episodes. If your spouse has a problem with pornography, resolving the issues can take months or even a few years. If you are willing to embark on this journey together, there is hope. Many couples have overcome problems with pornography in their marriage. They develop a happier relationship while also liberating themselves from unhealthy patterns in their lives. As you move forward, don't allow the past to hold the future hostage.

Additional Readings

Several prominent authors on the subject of boundaries and codependency include: Pia Mellody, Beverly Engel, Melody Beattie, Charles L. Whitfield, John and Linda Friel, Earnie Larsen, Robert Subby and Anne Katherine.

Notes

1. Mellody, Pia, et. al. HarperCollins, New York, NY. 1989.

2. Katherine, Anne. *Boundaries, Where You End and I Begin*. Fine Communications, New York, NY, 1991.

3. Robert Subby, "Inside the Chemically Dependent Marriage: Denial and

Manipulation," in *Co-Dependency: An Emerging Issue* (Hollywood, FL: Health Communications, 1984), 26.

4. Engel, Beverly. *The Emotional Abused Woman: Overcoming Destructive Patterns and Reclaiming Yourself.* Ballantine Books, 1990.

SECTION 2:
Disclosing Pornography Problems

7. The Choice to Disclose

In this section we have chosen to address the partner participating in addictive behaviors directly. Nevertheless, it is important for both spouses to understand what is at stake. The principles discussed here will help bring about disclosure—the first critical step towards reconciliation and change. Full disclosure is a choice made by the partner whose use of pornography is affecting the marriage. Even after confrontation, disclosure is still a necessary step. Being confronted with a partner's awareness of certain secretive behaviors and openly and honestly discussing the extent of those behaviors are two very different things. This information will help clarify the importance of disclosing secrets to a spouse and other individuals in your support system. The process of developing healthy strategies for carrying out an appropriate and effective disclosure plan will also be addressed.

Fear of Disclosure

You may be wondering if your issues with pornography are really all that bad or if they warrant open discussion with your spouse. Most men struggle with these questions, but after careful soul searching and introspection they recognize the importance of disclosure. If you are uncertain, consider how many times you have attempted to abandon your behaviors unsuccessfully. Do you lie to maintain your secrecy? Do you feel shame and guilt from living a "double life?" Are you isolating yourself and withdrawing from relationships and people? Are other aspects of your life suffering because of your inappropriate behavior? (See Appendix C for additional questions.)

If your answer to these questions is predominantly "yes," your compulsive habits will become more damaging and hurtful if no intervention is made and they are not stopped. Disclosure is a critical step towards healing and freedom.

Many individuals struggling with pornography problems want to tell their spouses. They fear, however, that their disclosure may place the marriage at risk. Studies indicate the majority of marriages stay intact if both partners are willing to work through the problems together.

Some people rationalize procrastinating a disclosure because they want to avoid hurting their spouses. This ignores the fact that dishonesty is as serious as the behavior itself. Avoiding hurting a spouse can simply be an excuse to protect oneself from a spouse's reaction and the consequences of one's behavior. As a result, many individuals choose to continue indulging in pornography while keeping it a secret.

Unfortunately, many spouses eventually discover the problem anyway. Then, the disclosure is usually forced and unplanned, and the spouse is unprepared to receive the information about the behavior. This can be disastrous, as in cases where an individual is fired for inappropriate behaviors on the job, arrested by the police, or exposed by the media. Disclosure forced by these situations is often incomplete and even dishonest because the participating spouse is trying to control the damage instead of having emotional honesty in the relationship.

If your life has not become what you had hoped, it is never too late to change. You can make changes that will bring a sense of peace that comes from being open and honest with your spouse.

Keeping Secrets

Secrecy and lies are the lifeblood of compulsive sexual behaviors. Disclosure breaks through the secrecy and may be your first step in the healing process.

Maintaining a secret draws energy from the relationship and requires a complex orchestration of lies. Time is wasted constructing lies to cover secrets and figuring out how to articulate the lie. In some situations, evidence is fabricated to substantiate lies. Perpetuating the dishonesty can require the individual to conform his behavior to the lie he has created. Additional lies are then necessary to cover up existing lies. Time is spent worrying if the lie was believed. Remembering the trail of lies can be exhausting.

Honesty and truth free all the energy used to maintain the secret and can provide a sense of relief for the person disclosing. Thus, many individuals report how liberating disclosures can be. In fact, even some wives report that their husband's disclosure, although painful, gave them a sense of relief. Hearing the truth provided validation that their suspicions and fears were not based on their own insecurities or distorted thoughts but on real facts and events.

Why Disclose?

The prospects of disclosing your sexual improprieties to your spouse can truly be frightening. Disclosure is a bold move that will affect your marriage, your children, perhaps even your social standing, and possibly your employment. There will be strong feelings, hurt and pain, fear and uncertainty. But there will also be freedom from the burden of living a lie, freedom from the guilt of betraying your spouse, freedom from betraying yourself, your hopes and aspirations. Why disclose? It may be the only way to gain any sense of health in your life, any real intimacy and trust in your marriage. And it may restore a sense of self respect.

Perhaps your need is practical: you may find yourself in a situation where you have no choice because your spouse is going to find out anyway. Regardless of the reason, disclosure is clearly the right thing to do. One study revealed that over 90% of spouses who received a disclosure felt it was the right thing despite the pain it caused them.[1]

There are certain compelling reasons to disclose. If a pregnancy results from an extra-marital affair or if sexual behavior outside the marriage has been unprotected, exposing the non-participating spouse to health risks such as HIV or other sexually transmitted diseases, disclosure is a must. Many spouses consider these risks to be the ultimate form of selfishness because they threaten their very lives. Although the impact on the relationship resulting from this type of disclosure may be very difficult, it is the right thing to do regardless of the outcome.

When you disclose, you will find the following recommendations helpful:

1. Talk to a therapist or church leader first so you have a system in place to support you through the process. You don't have to go through this disclosure by yourself.

2. Realize that fear is normal for people in your position. It's okay to feel this way.

3. If your goal is to get help, part of that process requires breaking the secrecy that fuels the behavior. It also brings an end to the denial.

4. Remember that over 90% of spouses want to know. Furthermore, 96% of spouses who disclosed report later that it was the right thing to do. Ironically, those who choose not to disclose in order to keep their marriage from falling apart ignore the reality that their behavior is bound to create emotional distance in the marriage. This may destroy the marriage they are trying to salvage through secrecy.

5. Disclosure will bring relief for you from the secrets you've been living. Most individuals report a huge burden lifted from their shoulders after disclosure. The shame and guilt will begin to lift as you replace them with truth and authenticity.

6. Although your spouse will most likely experience a range of strong emotions, she will also be relieved to know the truth.

7. The consequences you fear are a necessary part of the healing process. In fact, the pain you feel through this process will serve as a reminder to facilitate the changes you want to make.

8. Regardless of what decisions your spouse makes in response to your disclosure, you are doing the right thing by taking the first step toward developing healthy intimacy in your life.

9. If you choose not to disclose, there is a high probability your spouse will eventually find out. If the disclosure is forced at that point, the consequences will usually be more severe than if you take the initiative to disclose.

10. Remember that the decision not to disclose isn't about protecting your spouse. It's an excuse you use to protect your own emotions from your spouse's reaction.

Disclosing your secret behaviors will not be a painless process. It may be one of the most difficult decisions you ever make. Prolonging it will not make things easier. Every day you procrastinate disclosing is a day you could be working on your own recovery. It's a day that could be devoted to developing a healthier perspective or rebuilding the trust in your marriage. Have faith in yourself and in your spouse. Trust that the burdens you carry will be lifted by doing the right thing regardless of the outcome. If you are willing to reach out for help, there will be people willing to support you and stand by you when things get tough. Know that disclosure will change your life for the better and that the experience is something you can survive.

Notes

1. Schneider and Corley. *Journal of Sex Education and Therapy* 24:177-187, 199.

8. The Disclosure

People who have disclosed their secrets and revealed embarrassing or shameful information about themselves report that it has been a difficult and daunting task. However, they also report that it is an essential step on the road to healing and recovery. Their experience, both good and bad, has produced some helpful information about making appropriate disclosures. Their suggestions include the following:

1. Take a Personal Inventory.

Take a complete inventory of all your secret behaviors. Over the course of a few weeks, you may want to keep a note pad in your pocket and jot down inappropriate behaviors as you remember them. List the various thinking errors you have used to rationalize your behavior and the lies you've told to cover up your activities.

2. Categorize.

Create an outline and categorize your behaviors. For example, viewing pornography and masturbation are two different behaviors. Perhaps you have had several sexual affairs. They would be listed in their own category. Another category would be dishonesty, where you will list all of the lies you've told your spouse or others in order to hide your activities.

3. Get Feedback.

Present your outline to your therapist or members of your support group for feedback. Let them ask questions. These may be similar to the questions your spouse may ask. Don't get defensive at the reactions you get. Be specific and do not minimize your description of these events. For example, instead of reporting "I looked at pornography a few times," a more honest disclosure would be, "I looked at pornography 15-20 times over a one-month period. Each incident lasted between 30 and 45 minutes." You may not get this specific with your spouse, but it's important that you disclose responsibly by demonstrating an honest accountability of your behavior without any attempts to minimize. You may want to write down the questions asked of you and prepare appropriate responses in case your spouse asks the same questions.

4. Prepare Your Spouse.

If you are seeing a therapist, have your spouse meet with the therapist so she can be prepared for your disclosure. The therapist will ensure that she has a support system in place and also help you determine what timing would be most appropriate for the disclosure. Preparation can also include planning to disclose at the right time and place.

5. Write Your Disclosure.

Write down what you want to say and how you want to say it. Read it to your therapist or support group and invite additional feedback. Your comments shouldn't blame other people or things as excuses for your behavior. This disclosure will be a condensed description of your behavior without all the specific details. For example, if your disclosure included using pornography while masturbating, you would not go into the details about how you masturbated, what your specific fantasies were while you were masturbating, or what the actors in the pornography were doing. Help your listeners have an understanding about the frequency, duration, longevity, and severity of your behaviors. Avoid using statements that invoke sympathy or make excuses for your actions such as, "I was under a lot of stress." This written disclosure is to inform your spouse about your inappropriate behavior. It should not include language that requires or requests forgiveness because the focus is on your behavior. It is not intended to elicit behavior from her. (See the disclosure example below.)

6. Prepare for Reactions and Prevent Relapse.

You should have a plan to manage your own emotional reactions after the disclosure. Prepare yourself emotionally for your spouse's reaction. It may be negative. Do not get defensive if your spouse gets angry. Generally, the non-participating spouse needs to have her strong emotions validated, not suppressed. She has good reason to feel emotionally charged after hearing your disclosure. This may lead you to indulge in self-pity. You may feel depressed or hopeless. You may even attempt to escape this pain by returning to your addiction. Prepare in advance to prevent relapse.

7. Present the Disclosure.

As you present your disclosure, be aware that if you experience strong emotions during your disclosure, it can have both positive and negative effects. Crying, for example, may suggest you feel remorse for your behavior. It can also detract from the message you are trying to communicate by changing the focus of the disclosure to your remorse rather than your spouse's emotions, which need to be validated. Having self-awareness of your emotions is therefore critical to avoid engaging in tactics that elicit sympathy and therefore manipulate your partner's emotions. Your spouse may feel the need to focus on your emotions rather than on her own. Reading your disclosure while maintaining some eye contact is preferable because it will keep you focused and avoid straying from what you had prepared to say. Some clients prefer to disclose outside the office of a therapist. If you choose to do this, it would be wise to have an appointment scheduled immediately following your disclosure so support can be offered to both you and your spouse.

8. Answer Questions.

Part of your disclosure should invite your spouse to ask further questions. Be prepared to answer her questions without getting defensive. If you aren't sure how to answer a question or are uncomfortable with a question, you may request time to consider how you would like to respond. If you have planned the disclosure, you should be prepared for the majority of questions.

9. Accept Consequences.

Your spouse may choose to impose consequences immediately following your disclosure. For example, she may indicate that she wants some time to consider this situation and would prefer that you didn't stay at home for a few days. Respect this. Although your biggest fear may be rejection and abandonment, keep in mind that if you try to control or manipulate the situation to avoid negative consequences, your spouse may become resentful. You have had considerably more time to prepare for this disclosure than she has. Give her the time and space she requires. Remember, part of being responsible includes accepting consequences instead of avoiding them as you have done in the past.

10. Report.

After your disclosure, you should report back to your source of support. This may be a sponsor if you are part of a twelve-step support group for sexual issues, or it may be a church leader. Don't expect your spouse to provide emotional support for you. She will be trying to make sense of what has happened as well as understanding her own feelings and will most likely be unavailable to validate your emotions. As you report and think about your disclosure, realize that many offending spouses report mixed emotions. They may feel sadness because they witness first hand how much their behavior has hurt their spouse. They also report a great feeling of relief that comes from having the burden of their secrecy and lies lifted. While disclosure is a painful experience for your spouse, over 90% of spouses later report that the disclosure was the right thing to do. Time and space will allow the healing process to take place.

An Example

The following is an example of a disclosure letter written by a client to his spouse. This letter was not mailed; it was read to her in the presence of his therapist. A letter of this nature can be used as a guideline for disclosure to ensure that all the necessary information is disclosed and also to help keep the discussion focused.

Dear Rebecca,

I am writing this letter to disclose my inappropriate behavior. Through my own selfishness, I have indulged in activities that represent a lack of caring and respect for you and the children. These activities include pornography, masturbation, unprotected sexual relations with prostitutes, and intentional dishonesty to avoid being caught engaging in these behaviors. I have tested negative for sexually transmitted diseases; however, I encourage you to get tested for your own protection.

Although I may never fully understand how much I have hurt you, I imagine some of your feelings may include anger, hurt, disappointment, frustration, betrayal, confusion, rejection, hopelessness, and fear. You have every right to feel all of these emotions and more. Regrettably, I dismissed any thoughts about your feelings so I could rationalize my own distorted thoughts and convince myself it was okay to intentionally make choices I knew were wrong.

Even though I chose to indulge in these behaviors, I am not free to choose the consequences for my actions. I want you to have all the information you need to make decisions about the future. I am willing to disclose any additional information about these behaviors and also answer any other questions you may have.

Brian

Cleaning the Wound

Often, people attempt to abandon the behavior and recommit themselves to the relationship thinking they can bypass the important step of disclosure. This simply doesn't work. It's like placing a bandage on a cut filled with dirt without first disinfecting and cleaning the wound. Yes, the disinfectant hurts. There is pain involved, but the sting is a necessary part of helping the wound heal without getting infected again. If you don't go through the full disclosure process, the wounds won't heal. In fact, the infection that can result from covering your secrets may be worse than the initial problem.

In time, you may reflect on this experience, as others have, as one of the pivotal moments in your life, not because it is a shining moment but because you had the courage to break the cycle of secrecy and do what was right.

Timing and Method for Disclosing

The right timing to disclose is usually sooner than later. The method for the disclosure is also important. For example, the best time and place to disclose is not in a restaurant while on a date with your spouse.

Delivering a disclosure by phone, letter, or email is not appropriate. Such disclosures are irresponsible and attempt to avoid consequences that are part of being accountable.

There are very few circumstances where a disclosure should be delayed. However, there are a few situations that may justify a temporary delay. One rare exception was a client who began treatment and indicated that he had to disclose something that would involve legal authorities and eventually his own arrest. His interest in child pornography had escalated far beyond what he had ever imagined. He asked if he could have a few weeks to get his financial affairs in order so his family could be taken care of before he disclosed all the details of his crimes. After taking precautions to ensure that no one else would be victimized by this individual, his therapist determined he would have the needed time before he provided a full disclosure of his illegal activities. In this case, the timing was chosen to ensure the financial safety of his own family. He did disclose all the details of his crimes to his therapist and then to his wife shortly thereafter. The information he shared was devastating and would ultimately cost him his marriage. He was arrested and sentenced to prison. When later asked if he would disclose again if the time clock could be rewound, he indicated that although he was behind bars, his disclosure had given him more freedom than he'd ever experienced in his life.

The timing and method of disclosure may be best orchestrated in the safety of a therapist's office where an environment of support exists not only for you but also for the person receiving the disclosure. In the previous example, the wife desperately needed a safe place and support after the disclosure.

The timing and method of disclosure should take this into consideration.

Additional Disclosures

In an ideal world, disclosures should be as complete as possible the first time. Experience shows that disclosures made over a lengthy period of time can cause increased damage to marital relationships. They create additional obstacles for repairing the relationship by increasing distrust and prolonging the healing process.

Disclosure is often viewed as an event rather than a process. There are some circumstances that warrant additional disclosures. Dr. Jennifer Schneider and Dr. Deborah Corley suggest several reasons for additional disclosures:

1. The behavior has been so extensive and deception so widespread that the person disclosing genuinely does not remember everything that should have be disclosed initially.

2. The person acting out was under the influence of drugs or alcohol while acting out and doesn't remember all of the details.

3. Events considered insignificant initially are reconsidered as important during the process of therapeutic treatment.

4. The therapist recommends withholding information for a later time in order to prepare the receiver for the additional disclosure. In some cases, there may be a perceived threat of physical violence that requires additional time to work out the remainder of the disclosure. Generally, when a woman has to disclose to her husband inappropriate behaviors such as online affairs involving cybersex or real life encounters of sexually acting out, she is at a greater risk for an adverse reaction than if a man were disclosing to his wife. If a therapist perceives this risk, he may want some extra time to facilitate the complete disclosure.

5. If there are additional slips or relapses after the initial disclosure, additional disclosures will be necessary. Thus disclosure becomes a process rather than an event.

6. Limited detail may truly be all that the individual is capable of disclosing.[1]

A Final Thought About Disclosures

Following the principles outlined in this chapter will increase the likelihood that you will have an appropriate disclosure with your spouse. Keep in mind that any information about secret behaviors will be difficult for both you and your spouse to discuss. Remember that the disclosure is a process, not an event. Dedicate the necessary time to prepare properly. Be committed to becoming healthy. Be sincere, be genuine, and above all else, be honest.

Notes

1.   Schneider and Corely. *Disclosing Secrets: When, to Whom, and How Much to Reveal.* Gentle Path Press, Wickenburg, AZ. 2002, 68-69.

9. After the Disclosure— What Now?

A disclosure will elicit a wide range of reactions for you and your spouse. It is important to realize each spouse will interpret the disclosure differently. Both may feel the same emotion but for completely different reasons. For example, the disclosing spouse may feel relief not having to live a lie anymore. He is free from the burden of maintaining the secrecy. The spouse receiving the disclosure may also feel relief. Perhaps her suspicions have been validated. She doesn't have to wonder if she's imagining things anymore. Her thoughts and feelings haven't betrayed her and her intuition has proved correct.

Although the non-participating spouse may feel relief, she will mostly likely experience a wide range of strong emotions. As you read the following list, consider why a non-participating spouse would feel any of these emotions: anger, betrayal, rejection, confusion, depression, disappointment, fear, guilt, responsibility, frustration, despair, abandonment, rage, disgust, indifference, denial, helplessness, hopelessness, bitterness, resentment, powerlessness, discouragement, loneliness, uncertainty, doubt, hesitancy, devastation, distrust, worthlessness, suspiciousness, alienation, feeling victimization, humiliation, and anguish.

As you contemplate each of these emotions, you may begin to realize the damage your behavior has caused. You may want to fix or repair this damage. However, your spouse may not want to rely on you for her emotional support. Furthermore, you may want validation that your disclosure was the right thing to do, and yet your spouse is most likely dealing with her own emotions and unable to provide that validation. You will be tempted to personalize this rejection in a way that compounds your existing toxic (unhealthy) shame and guilt. This is where outside support is helpful. In the past you've most likely attempted to avoid these feelings through your self-medicating behavior. Although this may have provided temporary relief from your pain, this form of escape ultimately makes problems worse. The negative feelings you may be experiencing are part of the consequences of your behavior. If you act out as an attempt to escape the pain of these consequences, you avoid the accountability and responsibility that is part of your healing process. Remember, pain facilitates change.

Your spouse will most likely have many questions regarding your disclosure and she needs to feel that you will be open and willing to discuss her concerns. Don't get defensive about her questions and don't lie. If you're not sure how to answer a question or you're uncomfortable with a question, say so. It's not inappropriate to say, "I'd like some time to consider how to best answer that question." You may want to process these questions with someone such as a therapist and then report back to your spouse.

Experiencing Feelings—The Good, The Bad, The Ugly

Part of your recovery will require reconnection with your authentic self—your true feelings. Although the feelings you experience may be awkward or uncomfortable, learn to let these feelings flow through you rather than avoiding them. Part of their power to influence you comes from the way you interpret them, the amount of attention you give to them, and your reaction to them. Be content to sit and experience uncomfortable emotions. They are a part of you, and you will survive the experience.

Because you may feel guilty and responsible for your spouse's emotions, you may want to fix her pain. Realize, however, that this may be an attempt to minimize her reaction so you don't have to deal with her negative emotions. This may actually be an attempt to minimize your guilt and shame. Ask yourself if this is more about protecting your own emotions than about concern for your spouse.

It will take strength on your part to allow your spouse to experience the full range of her emotions without trying to dismiss them. When a person cries, for example, we are usually inclined to give them a handkerchief or a tissue. Why do we do this? Is this an attempt to stop them from crying because *we* feel uncomfortable? Do we interpret emotional tears as a bad thing? Dr. William Frey II, research director of the Ramsay Dry Eye and Tear Research Center in St. Paul, Minnesota, has studied tears for many years. In his research, he discovered that tears contain some of the same hormones that our bodies release during stress. The implication is that tears released through crying represent the body's natural way of releasing the stress hormones in our systems.[1] In this regard, emotional tears are a very healthy thing, and yet many people try to shut down crying because it's uncomfortable for them. Don't! Allow your spouse to cry, vent, and express her emotions. Don't try to stop them. What is important is that you validate these emotions. Don't avoid them through acting out or manipulating the situation simply to escape awkward or uncomfortable feelings.

Making Decisions—What About Divorce?

Couples working through a disclosure face a time of change and uncertainty. You and your spouse will have to make decisions. In some cases, couples consider the choice to divorce following a disclosure. Because a small minority follow through with this decision, it might be helpful to know that many couples who stayed together report they are glad they didn't make rash decision regarding divorce in the immediate aftermath of a disclosure. For them, their relationship got worse before it got better because in the early stages of their work together they were in a state of confusion and emotional trauma. It is important to note that the decision to stay in the marriage and work on the problems is contingent upon both spouses working towards resolving the issues in therapy.

Focusing on Changing Your Own Behavior

A disclosure is only part of the process of becoming healthier. It is important to realize you cannot control or change the way your spouse reacts;

focus instead on changing your own behavior. If your spouse decides to end the relationship or impose a temporary separation, you will need to allow her time and space to think about things. During this time you can focus on yourself instead of worrying about what she's thinking or doing. Changing yourself is something you do have control over. Ask yourself what changes and sacrifices *you* are willing to make. Change requires making specific goals and planning how you will achieve them. There are many questions to consider, including the following:

1. What puts you at risk for acting out, and what strategies do you have for relapse prevention? How will you permanently abandon and extinguish your unhealthy behaviors?

2. What changes are necessary to help rebuild trust in the relationship if your spouse decides she is committed to working through the problem with you? Would you be willing to agree to a polygraph[2] exam now and later in the treatment process?

3. How will you address any toxic shame issues about yourself (see Appendix E)?

4. How will you learn to develop healthy intimacy in your life?

5. How will you remain honest and open and thus break the cycle of secrecy and isolation? How will you be authentic and transparent with your spouse and others?

6. What thinking errors perpetuate your unhealthy behaviors, and how can you work towards correcting them?

7. What will you do if you have another slip? Do you have an understanding with your spouse about how any future slips will be disclosed? What information does she want to know if this happens?

8. How will you measure your success in recovery? Do you keep a journal?

9. What support systems do you have and how can they help you? Does anyone else need to be aware of your situation?

10. What elements will be part of your successful recovery?

11. What type of restitution is necessary to demonstrate your responsibility for your behavior? Have you disclosed to everyone who needs to know

(such as employer, church leader, or legal authorities if necessary)?

12. How will you develop healthy boundaries for yourself in the future? Do you have any codependency issues to address?

13. What are your needs and how will they be met appropriately?

14. What skills do you have and what skills do you need to acquire to become healthy? How will you learn the skills you lack?

Addressing each of these issues will take time. There is not one solution that cures all. Each answer will be individualized. Be patient with yourself and your spouse. Make incremental changes in your life—baby steps. Avoid blaming others for your problems and take responsibility for your own behavior. Accepting this responsibility also means accepting the consequences. This will take time. Resolving all the issues can take months and even years. Your success cannot be determined by the choices others make. Developing a plan, some goals, and a direction will help you feel at peace because you're doing things to correct the situation and make appropriate changes. This is something to feel good about. As one person said, "If you see someone on top of a mountain, you can be sure of one thing—they didn't fall there." Your recovery will require work and it will be an uphill climb. Trust that the rewards for your efforts will be there when you reach the top.

Conclusion

Disclosure is only part of a larger picture that includes your own efforts to become a healthy individual. This process requires more than just disclosure. Some of the elements of recovery are:

1. *Responsibility* must be taken for all of your behavior. This means that you are willing to own your behavior without blaming anyone or anything for your actions.

2. *Accountability* represents a willingness to disclose necessary information and admit responsibility for it.

3. *Disclosure* is the process of revealing appropriate detail about inappropriate behavior. Disclosure must be completed for true healing to occur.

4. ***Consequences*** for actions are accepted without complaint or defensiveness. This requires humility and responsibility. Some people are willing to admit they've done something wrong but take every opportunity to avoid consequences. Consequences aren't meant to be pleasant. They are often painful; however, the pain can facilitate positive change.

5. ***Remorse*** for the behavior shows true contrition and regret for wrongdoings.

6. ***Restitution*** requires making every effort to correct wrongdoings and undo harm caused by behaviors. Although it is difficult to make amends for some things, a good faith effort is made.

7. ***Abandonment*** of the behavior includes a resolve to keep trying, even if there are slips along the way. Never give up.

8. ***Recommitment*** shows your rededication to a life of healthy intimacy that includes being transparent and honest with your spouse.

We will discuss these concepts more fully in the next section of the book. When you accept the challenge to change behaviors that are detrimental to your marriage, it is easy to feel overwhelmed at first. But commitment to your own growth should remain foremost in your mind as you apply the principles outlined in this book. It is indeed possible to bring your behavior in line with what you know to be right, and as you work together with your spouse you will discover strengths in yourself and your spouse that you may never have known. By disclosing fully and humbly your previous errors, you can find an unprecedented peace within that comes from being open and honest with yourself, your spouse, and the other people you love.

Notes

1. Frey, William H. II. Ph.D. *Crying: The Mystery of Tears*. Minnesota: Winston Press, 1985

2. Although polygraph exams can be an important part of treatment, they should be suggested by the offending individual, not the offended spouse. Furthermore, it is important that as trust is reestablished that the non-participating spouse doesn't become dependent on the polygraph results. She ultimately needs to learn to believe and trust the word of her spouse again.

SECTION 3:
Abandoning Pornography Problems

10. Restoring Trust and Earning Forgiveness

Most women report that their husband's consumption of pornography constitutes cheating. Men, however, often see their behavior differently. One study indicated that less than 25 percent of men view such behavior as cheating.[1] This discrepancy often creates conflict around issues of repairing damage caused by pornography use. Additionally, the lies and deception used to hide sexual secrets can themselves have a devastating effect on marriages. Despite the seriousness of these ruptures in trust, husbands often downplay or minimize the significance of the impact of their choices and subsequently prolong the healing process. By neglecting to attend to the devastating consequences of their choices, husbands impair the restoration of healthy intimacy, trust, and forgiveness.

Listening to the Injured Spouse

After one man's wife asked a question about his behavior, he yelled, "Do we have to rehash this again and again?" Consider the function of this response. By resorting to anger, he shifted the focus from his behavior to hers. This tactic successfully enabled him to avoid responsibility for his choices. He may have temporarily silenced his wife's inquiry, but inevitably the repression of her confusion, pain, and feelings of betrayal will be manifest in other ways. She may begin to emotionally withdraw from the relationship. She may develop resentment which could be acted out in other, less obvious ways. Moreover, he has reinforced the pattern of avoidance and retreat that undermined his marriage in the first place.

Of course, the answer to his question—"Do we have to rehash this again and again?"—is, quite simply, yes. Until you adequately validate the impact your choice to use pornography has had on your spouse, you will find that the topic is likely to resurface again and again.

Husbands who frequently turn to pornography as a quick fix for coping with stress or challenges cannot expect to resolve the breech of trust in their marriage with the same "quick fix" mentality. This does not work. Impatience in restoring trust and healing is incongruent with the pace and nature of mature, loving relationships. Just as a man will need time to successfully abandon his pornography habit, a woman will need time to work through the process of being gradually open to trusting again—trusting that her partner will remain faithful, that her grievances will be addressed, and that she will not regret recommitting to the relationship.

Husbands, listening and validating your wife's pain is difficult. There is no question about it. But, your wife needs to know that you know how much pain she's felt, and this requires listening.

Listening is more than just nodding your head. Listening is being curious and asking questions. Listening is seeking to understand and see things through someone else's eyes. Listening means not getting defensive. Listening is an exchange of understanding where you gain insights and perspectives not previously held.

Consider the following account of a wife struggling with the discovery of her husband's pornography addiction. Try to see things through her eyes.

> It is hard to describe the exact emotions I felt at my own discovery of my husband's pornography use. The words *shocked, confused, devastated,* and *betrayed* come to mind. I felt as though my entire world was falling apart. I felt as though the very foundation of everything I held most sacred, namely my family, was being ripped out from beneath me. I cried every day for several weeks, couldn't eat, sleep, or concentrate. At the most random moments, my mind would envision what I imagined my spouse looked like while engaged in viewing pornography. These thoughts would leave me feeling sick to my stomach, and I

felt little motivation to do anything but the bare necessities for myself and my young children. Even though I was embarrassed by the fact that I had been "in the dark" for so many years, I also felt much relief in knowing I could trust in the instincts that had been telling me for some time that things were not right in my marriage.

Above all, I felt an overwhelming sense of sadness and loss. Some of the losses I most clearly felt included the loss of what I envisioned my marriage and family to be; a loss of trust in my husband; questioning my own self-worth (i.e. comparing myself to the women in the magazines, was I a good enough wife, etc.); financial losses (money wasted supporting his pornography habit); the loss of having a morally upright man in my home; and a loss of innocence (seeing and hearing about things I never knew existed in my conservative community).

One of the hardest things about the discovery of my husband's pornography addiction was the overwhelming sense of self-imposed isolation I felt. When your spouse suffers with this problem, it is generally not an issue that you feel comfortable talking about with your friends and neighbors. Although my religious leader knew about the challenges I was facing, attending church every week was very difficult because I felt we were carrying such a big secret with us wherever we went. Even having friends and visitors come over was very difficult for me during those first few months. When they would visit I felt phony, pretending that everything was okay in my life, because I felt there was no way I could tell them about the real issues affecting my family. I even made up excuses for a couple of months, telling my friends that I was really busy, but doing great, and apologized for not being able to meet. During this time I also requested to be released from my volunteer service in a leadership assignment I had for my local church. I didn't feel that I had the strength most days to hold my family together in addition to serving in my church. I volunteered to help out in the nursery at church, where I found bright, warm, welcoming smiles each Sunday, and I could avoid the painful "marriage and family" lessons in the adult classes.

This story is one of many and represents the tip of the iceberg. Unfortunately, this woman's husband was not willing to listen to her pain and the marriage was subsequently dissolved.

Women need to talk to their husbands and have their pain and frustration validated. If this does not occur, they find it challenging to be open to trusting again. Women report they do not feel safe. One woman asked, "How can my husband avoid making the same mistakes again if he doesn't understand how much he's hurt me?" These are valid concerns. In order for wives to feel safe enough to be vulnerable again they must have hope. They will find it difficult to be willing to risk if a husband won't even listen long enough to show sincere and genuine concern about their pain. When husbands refuse to be a witness to the devastation experienced by their wives, women have little confidence in the relationship and are left feeling hopeless about the prospect of change. Listening can be the beginning of an antidote for the pain and suffering caused by betrayal.

Restoring Trust

Restoring trust when fidelity has been breeched can be a daunting task. This breech requires that husbands be willing to develop insight and awareness about how this process works and accept responsibility to work on restoring trust. In this process, it is usually helpful if wives provide a road map so their husbands can have clarity about what they must do in order to repair damage caused by their choices.

It is important to differentiate between trust and forgiveness. Forgiveness is letting go of the right to expect a person to be punished. It means letting go of resentment, anger, or hatred. Trust is different. Trust represents confidence in a person's predictability. It is more than hoping a person will act a certain way. It is a firm belief that in a given circumstance a person *will* act a particular way again and again. It is the extent to which outcomes of a person's choices are predictable and reliable. It is possible to forgive someone and still maintain a healthy skepticism about their ability to behave predictably. Such skepticism may actually demonstrate an act of caring. Because individuals who habitually consume pornography will likely have a lifelong vulnerability to acting out, it would be wise to exercise caution and skepticism around circumstances or situations that might present challenging temptations to them. Consider the recovering alcoholic. He may have years of sobriety, but placing himself in harm's way by walking into a bar would be asking for trouble. Likewise, a husband may not act out using pornography for many years, but a wife would be justified in feeling uncomfortable about trusting him on the Las Vegas Strip. This limitation of trust is not about lacking forgiveness or about continuing to punish someone. In fact, a husband who has had vulnerability to pornography would be wise not to trust himself in certain situations. He should set boundaries to protect himself from circumstances where he might be susceptible to using pornography; taking precautious helps to restore the confidence of a wife who wants to be open to trusting again.

The most successful couples find concrete ways to ensure that the participating partner stays well away from danger areas. Clear expectations can be a road map to success. One wife complained that it was difficult for her to trust her husband's word that he would avoid danger zones since he had lied to her so many times before. How could she know he was where he claimed to be when she called him on his cell phone? This husband took the initiative and came up with a creative solution to his wife's concern. He purchased a set of cellular phones with video capabilities. Whenever she called, he would answer the phone with the video stream on so she could see where he was. It was a small gesture but it demonstrated his recognition that he had violated her trust and was committed to doing what was necessary to restore that trust.

Another husband realized that traveling with work responsibilities created tremendous anxiety for his wife. He had betrayed her confidence over several years of business trips. While on the road, he would frequent strip clubs, watch pornographic videos in his hotel, and had even solicited sex from prostitutes. His wife's devastation was overwhelming. She found it difficult to have any hope that he wouldn't act out while away from home. At first, the husband became defensive. He asked, "So what do you expect? Am I supposed to just quit my job?" After asking the question he realized that the answer in his situation was yes. He had violated the privilege of traveling with work, and in order to rebuild trust he needed to make a sacrifice that showed he was concerned for his wife and her feelings. In this particular case, the husband informed his boss that he could no longer travel with work and submitted his resignation. When the boss asked why, this man initially began to lie but found himself being frank and open with the boss about choices he had made while on the road. The boss was touched by this man's honesty and willingness to sacrifice his job for his marriage. He subsequently found the husband a different position in the company that did not require travel, allowing him to continue his employment. But, more importantly, his wife knew he was willing to make difficult choices to earn back her confidence.

As you work towards restoring trust you may be required to invest in small and simple acts, such as the cell phone intervention. In other cases, restoring trust may be more exacting, as in the case of changing employment. It often can require effort that feels uncomfortable or unpleasant or require changes that make you feel defensive or resistant. As Dr. Janis Abram Spring notes, "In choosing appropriate acts of atonement, you have to give the hurt party what matters to *her*, what *she* needs to trust you again. There's no formula, no prescription, for healing. . . . You may be asked to provide a significant intervention—not a few drops of blood, but a transfusion. It's better to err on the side of generosity."[2]

Earning Forgiveness

Webster's New World Dictionary states forgiveness is "(1) to give up resentment against or the desire to punish; stop being angry with and (2) to give up all claim to punish or exact penalty for (an offence)." Forgiveness, however, is not excusing or forgetting. A wife can forgive and still hold her husband accountable for choices he has made.

Earning the forgiveness of someone we've hurt is usually a long process. Many husbands lack awareness about what it takes to earn their wife's forgiveness. Healing a relationship hurt by betrayal takes a great deal of effort. It is hard work. It takes real commitment.

Dr. Spring suggests some of the following are necessary for forgiveness:

1. *Look at your mistaken assumptions about forgiveness and see how they block your efforts to earn it.* For example, some husbands assume their wives will never forgive them, so they don't try. Others erroneously believe that working to earn forgiveness implies they are the only ones who did wrong.

2. *Bear witness to the pain you caused.* Your wife can't heal until she is able to release her pain, and you must be willing to witness her anguish. Spring often says: "If you want your partner to move on, you must pay attention to her pain. If you don't, she will." In order to facilitate this process, initiate frequent discussions about the injury and listen with a caring heart.

3. *Apologize—genuinely, nondefensively, responsibly.* This involves making your apology personal, specific, and heartfelt. In order to apologize, you must know what you are apologizing for, and this necessitates the previous task outlined in bearing witness to the pain you've caused. Spring mentions several examples of bad apologies, such as the "lack of ownership apology which says 'I'm sorry your feelings are hurt.'" Other examples of bad apologies include the grudging apology, "I *said* I was sorry. What else do you want?" or the exaggerated, manipulative apology, "I hate myself for what I did. Can you ever, ever forgive me?"

4. *Seek to understand your behavior and reveal the inglorious truth about yourself to the person you harmed.* This involves exploring the sources of your behavior, including the values and beliefs that you abandoned in order to make poor choices. This may require you to examine deficits in your character, distorted ways of thinking, or lack of coping skills such as effective communication, problem solving, or coping with emotional pain.

5. *Work hard to earn back trust.* In addition to your sincere and heartfelt communication, your behavior often speaks much louder than words.

Your continuous and daily gestures of kindness and remorse will demonstrate that you mean what you say.[3]

Of course, there is no magic recipe for how forgiveness might be obtained, and each situation is unique. Each person has a different threshold. Some wives will be willing to work through infidelity, and others will choose to dissolve the marriage. Regardless, it is important for the husband to consider the factors that made him vulnerable to violating his spouse's trust in the first place and for both partners to evaluate what they will be willing to do in order for their to be real forgiveness.

Looking for a quick fix or brushing uncomfortable issues under the rug will not resolve the wounds caused by pornography use. Couples who work through these issues in a healthy way report that their efforts have provided a template for resolving many challenging aspects in their marriage. When proper healing occurs, couples discover a depth of intimacy in their marriage beyond what they've ever imagined. Both husbands and wives feel recommitted to their marital vows and a renewed sense of hope that their needs can and will be met by their relationship and their commitment to fidelity.

Notes

1. *American Sex Survey*, ABC News, Oct. 21, 2004.
2. Spring, Janis Abrahams. *How Can I Forgive You?* HarperCollins Publishers, New York, NY. 2004, 163.
3. Ibid.

11. Beginning the Process of Change

Although abandoning pornography problems may feel like a daunting task, many individuals have discovered reservoirs of strength beyond themselves as they've begun the process of change. Support from loved ones, skilled professional counselors, religious leaders, and close friends can be invaluable. Even with a strong support network, change comes with a price. It will require a lot of energy and effort. At times, things may feel like they're getting worse before they get better. Change will be emotionally draining and physically exhausting. Interestingly, some clients have said that giving up pornography wasn't as difficult as reorganizing their mind to a healthy perspective about sexuality.

Behavior modification is a complex process and many factors can potentially influence the choice to consume pornography. Similarly, many factors can influence an individual's choice to change. Perhaps a spouse has threatened consequences if nothing is done or a final warning from a boss at work regarding appropriate computer use in the workplace has instilled a sense of reality. Perhaps the husband arrives at a place in life where he has become exhausted and tired of living a lie, wasting time, and feels like his loss of self-respect and confidence isn't worth the price of using pornography anymore. Regardless of the catalyst for change, most find they are likely to vacillate in their commitment to abandon pornography. This is normal.

Feelings of ambivalence can lead people to believe their commitment to change is insincere. "Yesterday I really wanted to change, but today I'm not so sure." These types of thoughts can leave people feeling discouraged about their desire to change. In exploring this sense of ambivalence, husbands should consider the following categories of thoughts they may have about continuing or abandoning pornography use.

Perceived Advantages of Continuing Behavior

Despite a belief that pornography may be unhealthy, you must believe there is some benefit otherwise it wouldn't be so hard to abandon your behavior. Perhaps pornography represents a form of escape or a way of helping you relax. Maybe pornography is the way you cope with emotional pain, stress, or other problems in life. You may see your pornography consumption as a reliable and predictable "fix" and something you have control over. Many individuals indicate pornography helps them "disassociate" from reality and that it's "pleasurable." If you decide to change, these perceived advantages are what you will be letting go. It's important to recognize up front what you are sacrificing by choosing to change.

Costs of Continuing Behavior

Despite its perceived benefits, there are also costs associated with continued pornography use. Pornography can be an expensive habit, even if you get your pornography for free. It impairs healthy relationships. It contributes to a loss of self-respect. It is time consuming and contributes to a loss of productivity. Some individuals have lost employment or faced legal consequences because of pornography consumption. Multiple unsuccessful attempts to abandon the behavior can threaten self-confidence and leave individuals feeling shameful about their activities. Additionally, individuals typically consume pornography in isolation, which disconnects them from their partner and reality. A vast majority of individuals report their consumption of pornography is incongruent with their perceived values and beliefs. This can often lead to inner conflict or turmoil. These and many other costs associated with the choice to use pornography can influence the desire to change. But, to be certain, change comes with its own price tag.

Costs of Changing Behavior

Resisting cravings to consume pornography will be uncomfortable. If pornography is being used as a way of coping with problems and challenges in life, how will you deal with emotional pain in the future? It's likely you will need to develop new ways of confronting your stress or other problems in life that you attempt to escape through your behavior. This will undoubtedly require energy and effort on your part. What about the failed attempts at abandoning pornography and the impact this has on your self-confidence? If you try to change and have slips along the way you may feel like a failure. It may seem much easier to minimize pornography use as "harmless fun." This can happen when people believe that change increases the risk of further loss or suffering. You'll have to abandon such pessimistic thoughts if you're going to change. You might have to sacrifice some of your pride as you seek help from others to support you in your goals. This may be uncomfortable, embarrassing, or even humiliating! Professional counseling is generally helpful in abandoning pornography problems and this can be financially expensive. Are you willing to pay the many high prices associated with change?

Advantages of Changing Behavior

Men and women both report a variety of advantages to changing their behavior. Many make significant changes in their lives that involve much more than just abandoning pornography. Common reports include healthier intimacy; restoration of self-respect; increased confidence; decreased levels of depression and anxiety; increased productivity; elimination of inner conflict, guilt, and shame as well as feelings of congruence with values and beliefs. If all this sounds too good to be true, take some time and imagine what your life would be like if you weren't plagued by frequent cravings and urges to consume pornography.

As noted in the previous paragraphs, there is a wide range of thoughts and feelings people experience as they contemplate change. Remember that such perspectives are common and quite normal. You shouldn't be disturbed or derailed from your intentions to change just because you don't "feel" like changing every day. In fact, one principle of change involves taking one day at a time so you avoid becoming discouraged and overwhelmed by the many changes necessary to repair and heal the damage caused by the consumption of pornography. Although a broader perspective can be helpful, it can also be daunting when you realize how much further you have to go. It is better to focus on incremental change and what can be done today, as this is the most effective foundation for tomorrow's success. You will be tempted to indulge in self-defeating thoughts such as "Even if I resist today, my cravings will be worse tomorrow, so why try." Our reply is, who cares about tomorrow? You don't need to worry about tomorrow today. Just focus on keeping safe today.

One wife reported feelings of concern about her husband's ability to stop using pornography. She pressured him for a solid commitment. She needed reassurance that her husband would change his behavior. He humbly told her, "I can't make any promises about tomorrow, next week, or next month, but I promise you that today I will keep safe." Although her husband's commitment was less than ideal, this woman felt a burden lift from her shoulders. She reported, "I could relax for one day and not worry about him." Likewise, the individual who struggles with pornography problems will also feel a burden lifted if the philosophy of one day at a time is adopted throughout the road to recovery. On some occasions, you may even need to take it one hour at a time. The idea is to be present in the moment to moment details of your life and not entertain anticipatory anxiety about the possibility of falling short of your goals tomorrow.

Change is hard and requires a lot of energy and effort. It is likely that you will vacillate in your commitment to change. Such emotional rollercoasters should not be interpreted as a lack of desire to abandon pornography but a natural part of the process of change. Finally, adopt a philosophy of taking one day at a time. Don't fixate on yesterday's mistakes and don't create self-inflicted anxiety about the possibility that you could act out tomorrow.

12. Accurately Assessing Your Situation

It is important for couples to understand the complexity of thier circumstances in order for them to make appropriate decisions about the resources they will need to change them. One of the reasons professional counseling is often recommended for individuals with pornography problems is that there may be issues associated with pornography use and its effects on the relationship that are difficult for couples to see on their own. Another set of eyes—insight from someone you can trust—can be invaluable.

You may be tempted to judge your problem exclusively on the presence or absence of sexual behavior. This is a very narrow perspective. Research studies consistently demonstrate that individuals who have developed compulsive sexual behaviors often have other mental health issues that need to be addressed—issues such as depression, anxiety, social phobia, attention-deficit disorders, and concerns related to post-traumatic stress (often stemming from various forms of childhood abuse or neglect). Other characteristics common among individuals with pornography problems include tendencies toward perfectionism, proneness to shame, hypersensitivity, stress, loneliness, and a condition known as alexithymia, which is a deficit in the ability to emotionally identify, describe, or express feelings. Do you really feel confident in your ability to explore these types of issues with objectivity? A qualified professional counselor can help you explore these traits and offer meaningful ways to begin the process of change.

Before continuing, we want to clarify that we are not blaming a person's choice to consume pornography on mental health disorders. If any of these conditions exist, they are no excuse to rationalize acting out. We're suggesting that couples should be open to the possibility that there may be other forces at work contributing to their problems. If this is true, we hope you'll recognize and appreciate the value of additional resources that could be a great asset as you tackle the challenging task of modifying compulsive behaviors.

What to Expect If You See a Therapist

An assessment of your situation can be conducted in several ways. We will discuss what you might expect if you seek professional counseling. In Appendix B, we have outlined some considerations you might explore in choosing a qualified counselor. Even if you choose not to involve a therapist in your process of change, the following information might help you evaluate the variety of factors that might be influencing the participating partner's choice to use pornography.

The first session with a therapist usually involves exploring relevant history, evaluating the current circumstances, exploring details about the nature of your concerns and making educated guesses about what factors may be perpetuating the behavioral problems. When appropriate, a therapist may elect to assign a diagnosis, which is a label used by mental health professionals to describe a cluster of symptoms in a particular individual. For example, someone who is diagnosed with depression may have difficulty eating and sleeping, lack energy or feel fatigued, feel discouraged or hopeless about the future, and have difficulty making decisions or find it hard to concentrate. If you are using your insurance to finance treatment, a diagnosis is often used to collect a third party reimbursement. Despite the stereotypes that accompany diagnoses, these labels do not define people; they simply describe and categorize aspects of the symptoms people report.

After the first session, you might consider asking your therapist if they believe you meet the criteria for a diagnosis, and, if so, what they are considering. You have a right to this information, and if a diagnosis is applied to an insurance claim, you deserve to know which criteria a therapist has used to reach conclusions and any other relevant information related to the diagnosis.

Another benefit of diagnoses is that therapists can turn to the social science literature and see what other therapists have found helpful when working with individuals who have displayed similar symptoms.

One benefit of seeking help from licensed therapists is that they are trained to ask questions in order to uncover relevant information about the challenges you face. Each therapist works from a theory about how people develop problems and what factors influence human behavior. For example, some therapists use a cognitive behavioral approach to treatment while others may utilize an emotion-focused way of interacting with clients. Some therapists might evaluate your story in the context of the way you interpret life's events (sometimes referred to as narrative therapy). Narrative therapy is curious about what aspects of your story have been silenced and whether alternative characterizations of the *self* can be told. Depending on a therapist's perspective, they may place more or less emphasis on particular aspects of the information you provide.

The variety of approaches used by different therapists shouldn't disturb you. Decades of research have demonstrated that generally one approach can be as successful as another. The important thing is that you feel comfortable with your therapist. It is important that you feel safe and that you believe your therapist has the necessary credentials and skills to help you with your challenges. Working with a therapist will require vulnerability and risk taking, and if you don't feel like you will be able to explore painful aspects of your experience with them, you might consider a different therapist. Of course, it is desirable if you can find someone who has had experience working with issues similar to yours and, at a minimum, you should verify that the therapist is licensed in the state or province where they reside and that their license is active and in good standing.

As noted earlier, an interview will often explore your history. Therapists are curious about a vast array of items related to your life. For example, the environment where you were raised, your relationships with parents, siblings, and peers, significant life events (e.g. a death of a grandparent you were close to), how you preformed academically in school, extra-curricular activities, hobbies you enjoy, meaningful experiences throughout your life, and patterns of behavior you've adopted over time could be important factors in your treatment. We are also very interested in any issues related to sexual, emotional or physical abuse. We collect information about you in relation to your family and personal medical and mental health history. Such history might explore the presence of medical issues such as diabetes, cancer, hypoglycemia, or mental health concerns such as depression, attention-deficit disorders or anxiety. A careful history related to alcohol and drug use is taken. We explore any legal problems you may have had and how you perform in the work place. Educational background, attendance at college or a technical trade school or any other schooling after high school, marital status, your relationship to your children (if you have them)—all these things may be explored.

Your emotional experience is also an area of interest in clinical interviews. Therapists may ask such questions as: Do you feel lonely? How would you describe your self-esteem? What adjectives would you use to describe yourself? What is your greatest fear and what experiences bring out the best in you? On a more global level, we may ask about how you process emotions. Do you avoid awkward, uncomfortable, and unpleasant emotions? What do you look like when you're happy, sad, frustrated, or upset? Do you have difficulty talking about your feelings? Do others describe you as hard to get to know? When was the last time you cried? Are you a religious person? How do you define your spirituality? What accomplishments do you feel most proud of? What behavior do you most regret? How do you tackle challenges in your life? Is there congruence between your spiritual values and your behavior?

These are only some of the many questions a therapist may elect to ask. Of course, we also want to know what has brought you to our office. Why now and not six months ago or six months from now? In some cases, therapists use questionnaires, tests, or intake forms to explore these issues with you. In others, your therapist may desire to have a more formal evaluation. This might include other psychological testing that can provide information useful in helping you implement changes in your behavior.

Understanding the Bigger Picture

Part of developing a strategy for change is identifying factors that are associated with an individual's pornography use from a wider perspective. In psychology, this process is sometimes referred to as a Functional Behavior Assessment (FBA). Therapists seek to determine the "function" of a behavior and what influences might be antecedents or perpetuators. These assessments are designed to evaluate behaviors in the context in which they occur. Interventions (strategies for change) can be developed based on the various "ideas" an individual may have about what factors are influencing and perpetuating a particular behavior. We will discuss four aspects of FBAs below and give an example to illustrate how you might develop one.

Predisposing Risk Factors

Therapists look for factors that, when present, can increase an individual's vulnerability to engaging in particular behaviors.Growing up in a home where a parent used pornography, for example, could predispose a child being raised in that environment to also consume pornography. Sexual abuse and subsequent traumas could potentially predispose a child to developing dysfunctional behaviors related to sexuality.

There are also more ambiguous aspects of predisposing risk factors involving genetics. Although someone may not be genetically predisposed to developing a pornography habit, they might have hereditary tendencies that would predispose them to depression, a common problem among individuals who struggle with pornography. Mental health disorders can also make someone more vulnerable to pornography. For example, several research studies have found that some men with attention-deficit hyperactivity disorders (ADHD) also engage in hypersexual behavior. This doesn't mean that everyone with ADHD will develop pornography problems, but 26% of our clients are clinically diagnosable ADHD.

Another predisposing risk factor is a child's temperament. Anyone who has had a child knows that children come with their own hard-wired temperament. Some children are shy or timid while others are impulsive or rash.

Parenting styles can have an impact. Severe or harsh parenting, for example, combined with certain childhood temperaments can lead to depression in both adolescents and adults. If someone is chronically depressed, they are more likely to seek ways to escape their unpleasant mood. It is not surprising that during teenage years, such children are more likely to turn to sex, drugs, or alcohol as away of distracting themselves from their depression. Children who have highly reactive temperaments are more likely to suffer peer rejection, which can also lead to feelings of despair, failure, low self-esteem, loneliness, or shame—factors that precipitate dysfunctional, distractive or self-soothing behaviors. Of course, these factors also precipitate many problems other than pornography use (e.g. substance abuse, eating disorders, etc.).

Precipitating Risk Factors

Conditions or events that directly trigger acting out are sometimes called precipitating risk factors. For example, having a sexual craving or urge might directly precede consumption of pornography. Accessibility to a computer might be a precipitating risk factor for someone who views Internet pornography. Sometimes mood states such as feeling depressed or bored might be considered precipitating risk factors for individuals. It is important to note that some precipitating risk factors can also be perpetuating risk factors (see below). For example, family stress might precipitate acting out and the lack of developing more effective ways of coping with stress might perpetuate subsequent pornography consumption.

Target Behaviors

Targe behaviors are the behaviors that a particular individual wants to modify. They become the focus of attention and the target of interventions (strategies for change). Usually, there are multiple target behaviors that cluster together but one pivotal behavior which gives rise to the other actions. For example, if the pivotal behavior is masturbation to pornography, associated target behaviors might include turning the computer on, disrobing, locking an office door, and so forth. Generally, individuals develop rituals for acting out their target behaviors. These behaviors are all associated with each other and are carefully performed each time an individual acts out.

Perpetuating Risk Factors

Factors that allow target behaviors to be maintained are called perpetuating risk factors. For example, secrecy or denial about having a problem can perpetuate target behaviors. When present, these risk factors increase the likelihood that the behavior will be repeated. Reinforcement factors also perpetuate target behaviors.

The table on the following page (page 90) illustrates some of the items that might constitute an FBA for someone struggling with a pornography problem.

You might consider what *your* FBA would look like. Get out a piece of paper, divide it into quarters and begin brainstorming. Once you've identified items for each column, you can begin to conceptualize the origins of your behaviors and your particular risk factors. Next you might revisit the column of precipitating factors and rank the items that are most predictive of your pattern to act out. For example, maybe every time you face a deadline at work you find yourself acting out. Similarly, maybe you only *sometimes* act out when you're home alone.

Once you have created an FBA for yourself, you can begin to generate ideas about what steps you might take to interrupt precipitating risk factors, target behaviors, and perpetuating risk factors. You might evaluate your predisposing risk factors and explore whether it's possible to reframe issues such as sexual abuse or childhood neglect in ways that minimize their influence on precipitating risk factors. We will discuss developing strategies for change, including utilizing your FBA, more fully in the next chapter.

Functional Behavior Assessment (FBA)

Predisposing Risk Factors (Susceptibility to Behavior)	Precipitating Risk Factors (Antecedents to Behavior)
Dad used pornography (modeling) Mental health disorder Sexual abuse Childhood temperament Rigid or chaotic family system Childhood neglect or deprivation Emotional or physical abuse Traumatic experience Unhealthy boundaries Sexuality rigidity Attachment ruptures Genetics / biological factors Learned helplessness	Accessibility to a computer Isolation, home alone Boredom, loneliness Emotional pain or reactivity Attention bias Irrational thoughts Unintended media exposure Intrusive thoughts Sexual cravings, urges Feeling stressed Exhausted, tired Feeling restless Feeling anxious or depressed Flirting with temptation Unfiltered Internet access Complacency / apathy
Target Behaviors (Behavior Patterns)	**Perpetuating Risk Factors (Actions that Maintain Behavior)**
Withdraw from others Lock door, close blinds Turn lights off Turn computer on Compartmentalizing Disassociating / fantasizing Disrobe, taking clothes off Search for pornography Surfing TV channels Going to the video store Sexual arousal Placing hand on penis Masturbation / orgasm Neurochemical release Clean self, discard body fluids Excuse-making	Sexual orgasm, excitement Paired associations Not getting caught Secrecy and isolation Labels (e.g. I'm a sex addict.) Not getting help Denial about problem Work environment Pride (e.g. I'll fight this by myself.) No consequences No accountability / disclosure No social support network Media flooding Unfiltered Internet access Procrastination Dishonesty Minimizing the behavior

13. Developing an Effective Strategy for Change

People often attempt to develop strategies for managing pornography problems in the same way that they approach New Years' resolutions. They go from a complete lack of commitment to complete devotion and expect results to materialize miraculously overnight. Although there are some people who throw away their pornography once and never look at it again, this is the exception, not the rule. Most people find it takes patience and a willingness to work througgh good days and bad ones with a sustained commitment to improve Having said that, this chapter will explore strategies for change that have relatively high rates of success among real people struggling to overcome a compulsion to use pornography. As you read, keep in mind the factors and risks identified in your FBA from Chapter 12. Write down specific strategies that can help you as an individual or as a couple combat those behaviors. When you've completed the chapter, create concrete goals based on these strategies.

Again, it is important that both partners have realistic expectations about when to expect results. Change usually occurs gradually, and strategies to modify behavior should reflect that. Write your commitments down. Try to be sure that they...

1) are both structured and flexible
2) are expressed in positive terms
3) involve activities incompatible with the target behavior
4) are personally compelling
5) are realistic
6) are rewarding
7) are measurable

The most effective change strategies seem to have many or all of these characteristics.

Goals Should Be Both Structured and Flexible

People often establish very rigid and inflexible goals for themselves. In part, this may be a reflection of how desperately people want change. Goals structured in this manner simply do not accommodate the reality that all of us are human and things don't usually work out as perfectly as we'd like. All or nothing strategies should be saved for sports when you're down by a few points and the clock is running out—that one last shot from center court or "Hail Mary" pass into the end zone. In day-to-day life, however, each time you unsuccessfully attempt to change, it can reinforce negative behaviors. Failures are often translated into demoralizing beliefs about your ability to change—"I can't change because I've tried and failed so many times." Others convince themselves that "I'll never change because it's too hard." These types of internal dialogues can be very toxic. Certainly the self-talk we engage in will impact our ability to change. This doesn't mean you have to constantly whisper, "I think I can; I think I can," under your breath. It's okay to say, "Change will be difficult and challenging, but I believe it's possible if I'm willing to pay the price."

Accordingly, goals should be structured in a way that cultivates change but allows some flexibility so people are not left feeling hopeless about unmet expectations. It helps to structure your goals such that you can achieve some small victories early in your change process. This helps build momentum. You'll feel more optimistic about tackling some of the more challenging goals later on if you already have some victories under your belt. The following examples should help further illustrate this idea.

Example 1

Tom was consuming pornography both at home and at work on a daily basis. His first goal was to eliminate the presence of pornographic materials at the office to avoid loosing his job. He also made a commitment to lock his home office door if he chose to look at pornography at home so that his children would not accidentally walk into his office and see him. Tom's ultimate goal was to abandon pornography completely, but for the next 30 days, he practiced keeping these basic commitments that were realistic considering where he was at. They were not so rigid that Tom would fail. In fact, he was able to succeed on both counts and felt his sense of commitment grow.

Example 2

Greg continually lied to his wife in order to conceal his pornography problem. He made a commitment to be honest with his wife, regardless of any impending consequences. For the following 30 days, he reported to his wife every day whether or not he had consumed pornography. Hearing daily reports of his periodic binges with pornography was initially disturbing to his wife. Greg notice she would become emotionally distant each time he reported a slip. Despite these deficits, Greg learned that he could be completely honest with his wife. This represented incremental change. At the end of 30 days, he was still viewing pornography periodically. But Greg's commitment to honesty was a part of the change process. It was a real step in the direction of his ultimate goal and his wife came to appreciate Greg's ability to renounce deception as a sign of his commitment to her.

Example 3

Sally would meet men online in chat rooms. Conversations would quickly turn sexual. She would meet these strangers in motels for what she called "exciting rendezvous." Although she wanted to abandon this behavior, there was something intoxicating about these anonymous partners that was attractive to her. She wanted a reality check to help her wake up. Subsequently her first four goals were more oriented towards damage control or crisis management. First, she made a commitment to get tested to see if she had contracted any sexually transmitted diseases. Her second commitment was to carry a condom with her at all times. Her third goal was only to meet men in public places. Her fourth goal was to track how much time she spent in erotic chat rooms and find ways to serve in the community for an equal amount of time. These goals were short of what she really desired. But considering her ambivalence about change and her risky sexual behavior, it was a start.

Further, Sally recognized that her fourth goal about community service was on the ambitious side. So she gave herself further flexibility. If she wanted to reduce her commitment of service to 50% of the time spent in chat rooms this would be okay. Sally surprised herself in the coming month by reducing her time in chat rooms by 75% and spent her time instead helping out at a local charity organization that served abused women in a shelter.

Example 4

Brian had a goal to eliminate pornography from his life. But when he'd slip, he would feel that he had already ruined the day and give himself permission to act out as much as he wanted for the remainder of the day. Brian gave himself two goals. The first was to reorganize his beliefs about slips. He would stop measuring success in daily increments and begin tracking his success hour by hour. If he slipped in the morning, he would allow himself to recommit to change without feeling like the day was a compete failure. Second, he made the commitment to reduce his consumption of pornography by 25%. He kept progress charts to measure his performance and reviewed them after a month. On average, he had consumed pornography less than one hour a day. This was a 35% reduction. He also had several days where he had only acted out once. This was significant for Brian considering his history and background.

Although some might consider these changes marginal, they reflect the step-by-step process by which people really accomplish change. In each case, a standard objective provided clarity about what behavior modifications were expected while allowing enough flexibility to accomodate small failures. Subsequently the "all or nothing" mindset that so often characterized his previous attempts to abandon pornography was a thing of the past.

Goals Should Be Expressed in Positive Terms

Most people feel more empowered by positive statements rather than prohibitions. Consequently, you should be careful about the way you phrase your commitments. Instead of saying "I won't lie about using pornography," try reframing the idea using positive language: "I will be honest with my spouse about my day-to-day performance." The goal to "stop thinking about pornography" could be reframed to say "I will learn more about healthy sexuality and intimacy."

Sally used this principle when she developed the goal to serve in her community. Initially, she said she wanted to "stop being so selfish with my time by abandoning self-pleasuring activities." But she felt discouraged. So she restructured her goal about what she *could* do (I can serve in the community) rather than focus on what she *couldn't* do (I must stop being selfish).

Goals Should Involve Activities Incompatible with the Target Behavior

Another great thing about Sally's new goal was that she chose to replace a selfish act with a selfless one. This additional positive component turned out to be the thing that made all the difference in her performance. Because it is impossible to engage in two incompatible behaviors at the same time, goals that include behavior incompatible with the behavior you're trying to abandon are structurally more effective. In the other example, Greg's goal to be honest was incompatible with the secrecy that, in part, fueled his fantasies about pornography. Taken to the next level, Greg's goal to be honest might also have him take a closer look at the fraudulent message about sexuality contained in pornography. Greg might begin to contemplate the *self*-deception he practiced in order to rationalize acting out. As Greg becomes increasingly more honest with himself, he may well discover that consuming pornography is incompatible with a lifestyle characterized by honesty. He may well decide that being congruent with his values and beliefs is the most important thing in his life.

Former pornography users who have overcome their addiction are often found among the ranks of those working hardest to combat the effects of pornography on society. This may be in part because educating others about the harmful effects of pornography use is a dramatic way to work against the feelings and desires that might otherwise perpetuate their own former behaviors.

Goals Should Be Personally Compelling

A colleague of ours often encourages his clients to rapidly refocus inappropriate thoughts in order to avoid flirting with behaviors they are trying to abandon. However, when people refocus on something that is boring or mundane, these alternative thoughts usually do not have sufficient energy to lure thinking away from the intoxicating fantasies of pornography. Goals need to have energy. They need to be personally compelling. Consider the following example:

Kevin decided he wanted to finish building the basement in his house. Each day when he arrived home from work, he momentarily thought about his usual routine of going to his computer to look at pornography, but quickly turned his attention to the basement he was working on. This was exciting to him because he was creating something new. The basement had an element of novelty to it, and subsequently Kevin became passionate about the goal of rebuilding his basement. This goal redirected his attention to more productive tasks that, unlike pornography, left him feeling good about himself afterward.

From time to time in our practice, individuals will suggest that they don't feel passionate about anything but pornography. If this is genuinely true, then the first objective must be to find something interesting out there in the wide world. Past patients have discovered such interest as skydiving, art, music, family history projects, scuba diving, woodworking, and numerous others. Worthwhile distractions can be a secret weapon in the arsenal of those hoping to change their behaviors.

Goals Should Be Realistic

We have already discussed this at some length, but it bears repeating: When goals are unattainable, people usually become discouraged and give up. Many individuals have had so many unsuccessful attempts at abandoning pornography that they resign themselves to a state of hopeless. Some of these individuals begin to tell themselves, "This behavior isn't really that bad" or "Nobody is getting hurt from this." Even though they don't really believe these statements, they embrace these beliefs because the alternative would require them to admit they have failed at something they really wanted. Spouses who witness repeated failures on the part of their partner can also become discouraged and give up on the relationship. With so much at stake, it is critical to set goals that are attainable.

Care should also be taken not to flood oneself with goals. Don't decide to change five things about yourself all at once. It is noble to have so much ambition, but after a few weeks, you'll become exhausted and most likely start to let go of your goals. It's better to try one or two and achieve them than have several and achieve none. Also, it's completely permissible to take some goals for a test drive to see if they're a fit. Give yourself an interim period where you can see whether you're trying to do too much. If an interim goal doesn't work out or isn't a fit, it need not be interpreted as a failure because you're in the process of goal development, not goal implementation. Even formal goals should always be seen as works in progress. They should be revisited on a regular basis and revised as necessary. When goals are realistic, both spouses become more optimisticabout the process of recovery.

Goals Should Be Rewarding

Each time Kevin worked on his basement, he felt fulfilled because he was accomplishing something. It felt good to see his handwork take form. Sally found fulfillment in serving those worse off than she was. Another former patient turned to exercise and found that establishing a healthy lifestyle was an enjoyable way to strengthen mind and body while avoiding the temptation to be alone with pornography. These goals positively reinforced the continuation of the activities associated with the goal. It is ideal if goals can be set that have their own built-in reward systems. Some goals will have immediate pay-offs while others might take longer to be meaningful. Interestingly, pornography itself is the ultimate form of short-term pay-off. The long-term impact of pornography use is usually undesirable. Many individuals who struggle with pornography are impatient and intolerant of delayed gratification. This is why they turn to pornography for a quick-fix. If this is true for you, consider goals that have some immediate pay-offs.

It is also important to build in rewards for accomplishing longer term goals. If you achieve a chosen goal you might buy yourself something new or treat yourself and your spouse in some way. Rewards are a concrete way of commemorating success and reinforcing constructive behaviors. For example, one man decided if he could achieve 30 days of sobriety from pornography he would treat his wife to a meal at a restaurant they normally couldn't afford. The meal symbolized a small but significant accomplishment in their path to recovery. Similarly, another man decided after one year of sobriety from consuming pornography he and his wife would take a trip they had always wanted to take. Such joint rewards acknowledge that the struggle to overcome the affects of compulsive pornography use is a joing struggle. They validate the accomplishments of the recovering spouse while validating the patience and support of the other spouse.

Goals Should Be Measurable

Writing goals down and determining how they will be measured is an important aspect of goals. One goal, self-care, helps people feel better about themselves so they don't feel the need to turn to pornography as an escape from their internal emotional pain. Diet and proper exercise are one way of increasing self-care and are also incompatible with pornography consumption. One individual mapped out the following way of measuring this goal. Note, there should be a spectrum that allows you to track your progress on any given goal. For example, you might consider a scale and a description for each point on the scale based on the energy and effort you have invested in a goal each day. This way of measuring progress is illustrated below:

Goal: Improve physical health	Energy and Effort			
Monday	1	2	3	4
Tuesday	1	2	3	4
Wednesday	1	2	3	4
Thursday	1	2	3	4
Friday	1	2	3	4
Saturday	1	2	3	4
Sunday	1	2	3	4

1=*None*: Didn't exercise or eat healthy food

2=*Low*: Casual exercise and at least one healthy meal

3=*Moderate*: Half my exercise routine achieved and two healthy meals

4=*High*: Full exercise routine (vigorous) and three healthy meals

This goal is structured but also flexible (you still get points if you didn't do your very best). Also, someone could eat a healthy meal and still have an afternoon snack if they felt a craving to eat a treat. It's something the individual felt passionate about and also had a built-in reward system (he felt better after exercising and eating healthy food). It was realistic and not too rigid. The chart above was established as a way of measuring progress. After 30 days, the next chart was generated from the daily report of progress which gives an overview of the month's activities. Notice how the progress is not being conceptualized as all or nothing. There is a spectrum of energy and effort being invested each day and some days the individual does better than others. This chart can represent the first month of progress and a second chart for the following month can then be used to draw comparisons. In this manner, an individual can determine, on average, if progress is gradually being made over time.

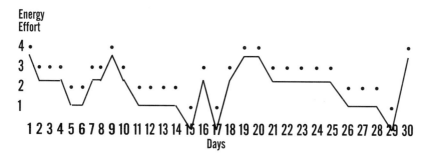

Summary

As you develop strategies for change there are several factors that can increase the likelihood of successes. These include establishing goals that 1) provide structure but permit some flexibility, 2) are expressed in positive terms, 3) involve activities incompatible with the behavior being abandoned, 4) are personally compelling, 5) are realistic, 6) contain some built-in reward system, and 7) are measurable. Revisit your FBA now and plan a few goals that fit into these criteria.

A schedule of revisiting goals and making modifications to goals as necessary should be an ongoing part of the change process. Finally, consult with others who know you about the goals you have set (especially your spouse) so you establish a system of accountability and reward yourself and your spouse when goals (even small ones) are accomplished.

14. Helpful Principles for Abandoning Pornography

Everyone governs their life by values and principles whether they are conscious of it or not. The principles that influence our behavior reflect the beliefs that we hold. In some cases, abandoning pornography requires recognizing your current beliefs and adopting new principles that will accommodate the changes you desire to make. Spouse's affected by their partner's compulsive pornography use also have to restructure their beliefs and commitments to determine whther or not they have the strength to be a support to the recovery process. More on this later. For now, we will examine some principles that others struggling with the effects of their pornography use have found helpful as they've worked through their respective processes of change.

Some of the principles mentioned in this chapter have been discussed previously in this book. We offer them again here as a reminder of their possible importance in your life and so that you might have a "buffet" of possibilities to help you overcome your vulnerability to using pornography compulsively. Pick up a pen and paper and write down the principles that could be helpful to you, and start creating a plan for how you will implement strategies to achieve the goals you have set as individuals and as a couple.

1. Be Accountable and Develop a Support Network

Part of taking responsibility for our behavior includes being accountable to yourself, spouse, and others. The pattern of reporting to others is a principle of positive change, because to some extent, all of us are somewhat externally motivated. Religious leaders, a spouse, trusted friends, and groups sponsored by mental health agencies can provide an invaluable network of support that cultivates the abolishment of secrecy and can actually increase your motivation to change. Individuals who participate in twelve-step programs for recovery might also adopt a sponsor to work with. Developing a network of support to which you are accountable is an integral part of recovery. Learning to interact with and rely on others is the antithesis of the isolating and disconnecting influence habitual pornography use can have. When interacting regularly with members of a support network, individuals may consider reporting the presence or absence of their behavior, steps they've taken to make positive change, and how they are meeting life's challenges differently.

Another benefit of reaching out to others is that such behavior is an antidote to loneliness. Loneliness has been directly correlated with pornography problems. When connecting with others, it is helpful to take risks such as being emotionally vulnerable and completely honest.

Support networks can also provide a cheerleading role when you feel tempted or challenged. They can offer encouragement and suggestions about strategies for change.

2. Take Responsibility for Your Recovery

Be careful, however, not to expect others to take responsibility for your recovery. This is something you must do. Therapists, religious leaders, your spouse, friends and others are not responsible for solving your problems. A man once asked his sponsor, "What should I do?" This wise sponsor replied, "What do *you* think you should do?" to which the man quickly responded, "I don't know." Then, this marvelous sponsor said, "Maybe you should go home and wrestle with that question and I'll spend some time thinking about it and then we can meet together later and talk some more." This sponsor understood the value of not being quick to rescue this individual or to give out advice without requiring some effort on the part of the person struggling to abandon pornography.

You develop a plan for your recovery and then take that plan to others in your network for support and feedback.

Another aspect of taking responsibility requires appropriate disclosures.

In particular, these disclosures need to be made to those who have been in-jured by your choices. Addressing the grievances of those who have been hurt requires effective apologies. This is not synonymous with being sorry you got caught. In order to offer an effective apology we must know the depth of the pain that has been caused. "I'm sorry for using pornography" is not an apology. It's not even close. You have to start by asking loved ones how your choice to consume pornography has impacted them. What has their experience been like? What aspects have been most painful? What losses have they suffered, and what was it like for them to feel so betrayed and deceived by someone in whom they had placed so much trust? If you really ask these questions with an honest desire to acknowledge your faults, you will start to get a glimpse of some of the things you will need to apologize for.

Many individuals avoid disclosure because they are afraid of the conse-quences. Some postpone disclosures because they're trying to have a period of time when they've refrained from acting out so when they confess their behav-ior they can report it as a problem of the past. The flaw in this approach is that a substantial period of abstinence is difficult to obtained. Weeks turn to months. Years go by and the problem hasn't gone away. Besides, retroactive disclosures continue the pattern of pre-meditated deception.

Another common practice is for an individual to disclose less severe problems, wait for the dust to settle, and then disclose more at a later time. For example, one man told his wife that he had been looking at pornography while at work. The couple worked on the devastation caused by this confession, and after his wife had processed the experience, several weeks later he reported that he had also been to some inappropriate establishments while traveling. Incremental disclosures like this are systematically destructive to relationships. You essentially condition your spouse to believe that they cannot trust that everything you say is completely honest. How would you react if a physician only partially irrigated your cut prior to providing sutures? You'd be concerned that dirt left in your wound might cause further infection, and you'd want the doctor to cleanse the affected area completely even if it caused more pain ini-tially. When you disclose, make sure that you give an accurate and complete report, providing those who need to know with the information they need to make decisions about the future.

As part of the process of disclosure, the one who has breeched the trust should initiate regular conversations, weekly and even daily if necessary, to update their spouse on the ongoing effects of their behavior—particularly when a commitment to recovery has been made. Don't get into the trap of avoiding conversations about your recovery just because your spouse hasn't brought the topic up. Trust us, it's on their mind. If you find yourself having difficulty tolerating discussions about recovery or you're hypersensitive when your spouse makes inquiries, then it might suggest you're not involved in a healthy recovery. Don't fear these conversations. Lean into them. It is these very fears you should be curious about. Do not seek to avoid them. Seek to understand why inquiries or discussions about your recovery seem uncomfortable or threatening. The tendency to say, "Things are going well, I don't want to ruffle feathers or stir up the pot," is really an excuse you use to rationalize and avoid emotional pain. "I don't want to worry my spouse," one man said. Another reported, "She's suffered enough, she can't handle any more." That's nonsense. You're trying to protect yourself from your spouse's adverse reaction and the consequences of your choices.

Be honest in your disclosures and abandon the habits of secrecy that have maintained the behaviors you're trying to change. Remember, secrecy is the lifeblood of pornography habits. Shame breeds dishonesty, and dishonesty breeds more shame. Every day you maintain a lie is a day you could be recommitted to cultivating honesty. Remember that most partners are equally as disturbed by dishonesty as they are by your sexual behaviors, and your deception will inevitably be discovered anyway.

A final comment about disclosures! The research is very clear that parents should *not* disclose details of their mistakes to their children. In several retroactive studies, children (even adult children) report they would have preferred that their parents would have not disclosed details. In many cases, they said it was tramatic for them. It is sufficient to say, "I've made some mistakes and I'm trying to make some changes in my life."

3. Take One Day at a Time

People can become discouraged and overwhelmed when they fixate on the many changes necessary to repair and heal the damage caused by their consumption of pornography. Although a larger perspective can be helpful, it can also be daunting when we realize how much further there is to go. This is a valuable lesson for recovery. Focusing on incremental change and what can be done today is the most effective foundation for tomorrow's success.

4. Consider the Small and Simple Things

It's helpful to focus on the small and simple things and not look for some great solution for your problem. Most individuals who abandon pornography do so gradually until they eventually let go and move on with their lives. Those who look for a miraculous solution often remain stuck. There are many small things we can do to modify behavior, but our pride and stubbornness can prevent us from doing these things, which may include daily self-affirmations, checking in with a sponsor, writing in a journal, getting some exercise, eating properly, or small acts of service to your spouse, other loved ones, or other people in greater need than yourself.

5. Establish Appropriate Boundaries

Those struggling with pornography should avoid any potentially compromising situations. An appropriate boundary might include placing the computer in an open area and having a family policy that requires any family members who are exposed to pornography to report it the same day. Those who successfully overcome their compulsive behaviors take pains to create environments that will keep them safe. A client in group therapy mentioned that the problem with seeing how closely we can drive to the edge without going over the cliff is that we assume we can see where the edge is—and that is rarely the case. Safety is found in establishing and maintaining healthy boundaries.

6. Eliminate "Hooks"

Hooks are avenues that provide a gateway for people to return to behaviors they're trying to change. Hooks maintain secrecy and isolation, which perpetuate pornography use. Eliminating hooks involves identifying and responding differently to triggers that precipitate acting out. Severing all "hooks" involves eliminating the things that could enable you to return to the behavior. Many people run from temptation but leave a forwarding address. Failure to eliminate hooks often results in finding yourself repeating mistakes from the past. Perhaps it's files on your computer that haven't been deleted or small lies you maintain and refuse to disclose. Maybe it's throwing away a list of ways to act out. You likely know full well what the hooks are for you. A client once commented, "You really have to be humble enough to do whatever it takes even if everything is not required of you."

For example, one man was leaving on a business trip. He knew being alone in the hotel at night was a risk factor for him. Subsequently, he called the hotel in advance and asked them to remove the T.V. from his room. This represented an intervention that removed a hook for him. It wasn't that he couldn't ever watch TV. In fact, he could watch TV in the lobby or in the exercise room of the hotel. These TV's didn't have pay-per-view pornography so he felt safer with these arrangements.

7. Develop Healthy Intimacy

Each of us must understand that healthy intimacy requires us to bridle our passions and that lust impairs our ability to love. In part, this is true because lust focuses on a very narrow aspect of intimacy—sex—and it promotes selfishness that erodes a healthy relationship, which requires *selflessness*. Pornography is the antithesis of a healthy relationship because it depicts a fraudulent message about sex and distorts expectations about physical intimacy in marriage. For example, pornography suggests women have insatiable sexual appetites and it minimizes the harmful effects of sexually promiscuous behavior.

Sexual union is a physical manifestation of intimacy between two individuals and can be symbolic of a far deeper bonding. Sexual union between a husband and wife is an outward manifestation of their inward commitment to connect more deeply as spouses. Sexual intimacy is an exchange between two people intended to symbolize a manifestation of their desire to renew their covenant of marriage and their commitment to each other. It is an opportunity for a husband and wife to become one by connecting and bonding with each other. During physical intimacy, our most intense physiological feelings are expressed and experienced, creating a powerful, paired association between transcendent feelings of pleasure and being connected with our partner. This, in turn, reinforces our desire to be close with them. Additionally, being naked with our spouse requires vulnerability and risk taking, which are traits of intimacy. The constellation of these principles is what should govern intimacy between husbands and wives, and pornography is the antithesis of everything that cultivates this type of relationship. It is a counterfeit that will never compare to true intimacy.

Some argue that erotica can act as an educational vehicle to help couples enhance their sexual intimacy. In such cases, the erotica referred to is void of many of the degrading or violent themes found in pornography. Even in cases where erotica is used, our experience in counseling couples is that usually one partner is uncomfortable with this approach. This can be discussed and explored provided it is done respectfully. Alternatively, most couples, with a skilled sex therapist, can explore their beliefs and values around sexual intimacy and also talk about what they would want in their relationship without watching erotica. In cases where someone has previously struggled with pornography, erotica may be a hook that would trigger someone to return to pornography use.

One reason we want to illuminate the topic of sexual intimacy is because one of the most interesting discoveries of many individuals who overcome pornography is that resisting the urges and cravings to act out is the easy part. The hard part is reorganizing their beliefs and perspectives about sexuality in their relationship in order to replace the many distorted messages they have consumed about sexual intimacy through pornography. Moment-to-moment interventions are what psychology labels first-order changes. Second-order changes, however, seek for a deeper, more meaningful influence.

Consider the man who finds himself in a boat that is sinking. He can pick up a bucket and begin to scoop water out of the boat. This is a first-order change. It will keep him afloat for a time, but he may eventually find himself exhausted. A second-order change would look for the hole in the boat and attempt to plug it so water would be prevented from filling the vessel. Second order changes include reorganizing beliefs about sexuality, relationships, or how to react to painful emotions differently. It is important to realize that abandoning pornography is not the end goal. Developing an understanding of healthy intimacy and leading a life that will cultivate such relationships is the more meaningful goal to strive towards.

8. Write Regularly in a Journal

Begin now keeping a journal. Consider keeping two journals. One is the journal you will keep to pass on to posterity. The other is a private journal that may eventually be destroyed. This can be your "therapy" journal where you give yourself permission to write anything that's on your mind. You can process difficult and painful emotions you may be experiencing as you work through recovery or talk about embarrassing or awkward thoughts and feelings. There is something therapeutic about the process of writing or typing out thoughts and feelings. Let this journal be a place of refuge amidst the storms you may face. Let it provide a forum for you to express your most personal thoughts in a brutally honest way. When the journal has served its purpose, feel free to destroy it as you move forward with your life.

9. Remember to Be Kind to Yourself

Learning the language of self-compassion can be as difficult as learning a foreign language. Positive affirmations that focus on progress should be identified and used. Self-talk that focuses on failure and hopelessness usually produces failure and hopelessness. Conversely, the opposite is also true. Self-talk that focuses on success and positive outcomes usually produces the same.

Prominent psychologist Albert Bandura from Stanford University has dedicated much of his career to studying self-efficacy as it relates to positive outcomes in treatment. *Self-efficacy* refers to an individual's beliefs about his competence in a particular area. It shouldn't surprise us that a belief about our ability to accomplish something is highly correlated with the reality of us accomplishing it. Unfortunately, pessimism is too prevalent in our society today. One man said, "I don't know who was driving the little train that said 'I think I can' but my train isn't on the same track, and every time I say 'I think I can,' my train gets derailed." This man's pessimism was self-destructive. He talked himself out of treatment, and out of a marriage he believed couldn't work. If he put as much energy and effort into confronting his pornography problem as he did in convincing himself he couldn't change, he would probably be in a different place now.

It is important to realize that being kind to yourself isn't letting yourself off the hook. Sometimes being kind to yourself requires firm love that may produce discomfort. But being kind to yourself involves doing things that will help you be your best self. Love usually produces better outcomes than criticism, and thus it is vital we avoid harsh self-criticism that is emotionally and verbally abusive to ourselves. Find a list of positive self-affirmations and recite aloud kind things to yourself every day.

Embracing fear, which is the antithesis of the faith you should have in your recovery, is also a form of self-hatred. Sometimes we don't try because we become paralyzed by fear that we will fail, and so we suffer further loss. This perspective perpetuates a "helpless" or "victim" mentality about our ability to regulate our reaction to sexual urges or cravings. It is more helpful to translate self-defeating thoughts to realistic self-talk. For example, instead of saying, "I can't," you might consider saying, "This is difficult and challenging at times, but I will continue to take one day at a time."

Being kind to yourself also requires you to take an inventory of your life and eliminate things that are adding unnecessary stress and chaos in your daily routine. Take some time for self-care, rest, and relaxation so you can have the strength you'll need to tackle the daunting task of working through the process of change. Change requires a lot of effort and energy, and when you're tired and exhausted you're less likely to invest the required work necessary to change. In company with this philosophy are the principles of proper exercise and nutrition. The United States Department of Agriculture has reformed the old food pyramid, and the new food guidelines can be found online at www.mypyramid.gov. Take time to familiarize yourself with the new recommendations and recommit to a lifestyle of healthy nutrition and exercise.

10. Learn to Discriminate between Guilt and Shame

Guilt says, "My behavior is bad." Shame says, "I am bad." It is okay to feel guilty for choices that have been made but shame thwarts the process of genuine recovery. It is a counterfeit where people feel they can somehow punish themselves for mistakes they have made and subsequently make things right. People beat themselves up, believing that because they feel bad they have suffered for their mistakes. Punishing oneself does not constitute restitution for choices that may have injured your partner or others.

11. Know You Can Survive the Discomfort of Withdrawal

Understand you can survive the uncomfortable cravings of withdrawal from your addictive behaviors. Some people are quick to interpret cravings as evidence of their lack of desire to change. This is a mistake. Even if your desires to change remain constant, your body will continue to crave the mood-altering experiences that it has been conditioned to expect. Although it may be very uncomfortable and unpleasant to withstand them, it is possible to survive the intense urges and cravings you feel for sexual gratification. In order to manage these cravings, you may consider appropriate ways to express sexuality or alternative activities such as exercise. Many religious subcultures practice periodic fasting (abstinence from food for a period of time; e.g. 2 or 3 meals in a row once a month) as a way of developing self-restraint. This practice is actually consistent with the mindset of surviving the cravings of withdrawal and has been helpful among many clients who have reported improvement in their ability to manage inappropriate urges.

Another aspect of managing feelings is a perspective capable of distinguishing the difference between "feeling good" and "feeling right." Just because something feels good doesn't mean it will feel right. Similarly, things that are right don't always feel good. Think of the bodybuilding motto: "No pain, no gain." Individuals who struggle with pornography problems often report feeling good in the moment but often say that after they've acted out they feel empty inside and feel what they have done isn't right. Some have claimed that the chief cause of failure and unhappiness in life is trading what we want most for what we want at the moment. This short-term tunnel vision can often lead to people feeling remorse and regret about impulsive decisions made without thinking about future consequences.

12. Watch Your Thoughts

What does it mean to "watch" our thoughts? The word *watch* suggests we evaluate, monitor, observe, analyze, and consider the variety of thoughts we (1) receive, (2) manufacture, or (3) entertain.

You have probably been told on numerous occasions to just stop thinking about pornography. A colleague has observed that in order to stop thinking about something, you must know what it is you're not supposed to be thinking about, and therefore you must think about the very thing you're trying to avoid. If this strategy hasn't worked very well for you, now you understand why. We'd like to invite you take a different approach: You ought to think a lot about pornography, but you need to think about it in a way that reflects the realities of your life, not your fantasies.

Consider what role or function pornography serves in your life. What needs are you trying to meet? What is at the core of your behavior when you act out? You may be attempting to meet a need to feel loved, desired, or accepted. One client commented, "Your favorite porn sites will never reject you." There is a theme of reciprocation in the fantasies of pornography that will lead you to believe that the actors portrayed want you just as much as you want them. What the viewer forgets is that it's an act, and in real life rejection is often more common than reciprocation. A recent study examined over 1000 men's sexual fantasies and found a single common denominator consisten to all of them. Each man reported fantasizing that they were desired or wanted by the object of their fantasy.

Alternatively pornography may represent an attempt to meet your need to feel adequate or appreciated. What thoughts or feelings precipitate your fantasies? A number of studies have revealed that individuals who have developed habitual pornography problems report more distressing levels of loneliness in their lives. Is pornography your attempt to avoid feelings of loneliness and feel connected or attached to someone? Perhaps your fantasies are an attempt to provide a temporary distraction or escape from unpleasant, uncomfortable, or undesirable emotions such as stress, anxiety, sadness, or discouragement. You may yearn to feel connected, validated, and deeply understood by another human being who knows everything about you and loves you anyway. But your continued use of pornography may have desensitized you in a way that impairs your ability to connect with others in meaningful ways.

Some people consume pornography to distract themselves from boredom or because they are seeking excitement, novelty, or variety in life. Some people get a rush from exploring the forbidden and taboo despite the fact that the sexually promiscuous lifestyle portrayed in pornography is anything but glamorous.

The point is that you need to begin thinking critically about the thought processes that trigger or perpetuate your pornography use. Be honest with yourself about what it is you're actually doing. There are several ways to watch your thoughts that might be helpful for you to know about.

First, we want to be clear that we're not suggesting that you should focus on the sexual content of your thoughts. That is, you have to be able to look beyond the sexual scenario, theme, or fantasy of the content. This includes avoiding mental imagery of sexual acts or the precipitating events that occur prior to acting out. What you want to evaluate is how you *appraise* such content. What meanings do you attach to it? Meaning refers to how we interpret a particular stimulus. What does the content represent or symbolize? Why is it important and what is the purpose of the thought? As already indicated, the thought content may represent an opportunity to escape uncomfortable or unpleasant feelings such as stress, anxiety, depression, sadness, or loneliness. It may symbolize a chance to feel accepted, desired, or adequate. It may stem from a desire to experience something pleasurable. The content may have importance as a way of coping with problems or as a way of soothing yourself in times of emotional pain. There are many assumptions that your interpretations rely on in order for the content to have pleasurable meanings in your life. It is important to be curious about what these assumptions are and to explore the accuracy of these perceptions against external evidence.

Next, as you evaluate the content, consider what psychology refers to as "attention bias." What aspects of your fantasies do you focus on, and what aspects do you ignore? How do you bias the content of pornography by attending to particular pieces of information while excluding others? For example, you might perceive the content as exciting or pleasurable while ignoring the fraudulent messages about human sexuality associated with it. Women in real life seldom have insatiable sexual appetites and rarely act sexually promiscuous without drugs, financial compensation, or other problems in living. The behavior depicted as harmless fun would inevitably result in unwanted pregnancies or sexually transmitted diseases. Imagine how excited you'd feel sitting in a medical clinic waiting for results from an HIV test. Clients say it's hell. These are the realities you ignore whenever you consume pornography.

When some people are periodically exposed to pornography, as we all are, their attention bias recognizes aspects of pornography that leave them feeling sad. These people see women depicted in pornography as degrading themselves. Others believe their lives are filled with tragedy and often include histories of abuse.

The third aspect of our thoughts you should pay attention to is how your thoughts reflect your more deeply held beliefs. Do you believe that a counterfeit form of sex can be a substitute for genuine, sincere, and authentic happiness found in the context of healthy intimacy? Do you believe that the payoff of acting on the thought is worth the possibility of incurring the consequences (e.g. upsetting your spouse or feeling guilty afterwards)? Do you maintain a belief that if an attractive woman would desire you or be pleased by you that this is the necessary criteria to validate you as a person? Would this make you feel better about yourself? Give yourself real answers to these questions—not just what you wish you believed but what your actual belief structure is.

The way you appraise the content of your mind, the information you attend to and ignore, and the meanings you attach to your thoughts reflect your underlying beliefs, which will ultimately influence how you feel. These feelings occur in *response* to or *concurrently* with the content of your thoughts. Feelings might include excitement, a rush, or nervousness about the possibility of being caught if you acted on the content of the thought (e.g. acted out sexually with someone other than your partner). Some individuals say they begin to experience a trancelike state where they feel detached or disconnected from reality. Pornography for these people occurs when they are disassociated from others and their environment. Some people report feeling ambivalent, caught between the desire to act out the content and their desire to remain congruent with their values or beliefs. Additionally, physiological feelings such as tingling, increased heart rate, a fluctuation in respiration, and sexual arousal occur creating intense emotion at the very thought of consuming pornography. What is important to realize throughout this entire process is that you are the one in the driver's seat. You can change your beliefs that have drawn you to pornography. If you don't like your beliefs, work on adopting new ones. If your attention bias is skewed in a manner that prevents you from being your best self, pay attention to different aspects of the content that comes into your mind. Get brutally honest about your thoughts and be curious about what you really need. Is it sex or something else?

13. Connect with Your Feelings

Some individuals suffer from a condition known as *alexithymia*, which is a deficit in the ability to process emotional experiences. Specifically it refers to the inability to identify, describe, and express emotions. Such people lack emotional awareness for themselves and those around them. Men are often accused of being more emotionally disconnected than women. There's the old joke, "What do men and mascara have in common? They both run at the first sign of emotions." Unfortunately we live in a world where men are often culturally conditioned to suppress their feelings. Sadly, it has become a sign of weakness for men to become emotional. Research has shown that men are actually capable of identifying their emotions more accurately than women but that they choose not to express their feelings as often, and so it has been assumed that men are emotionally unaware. The next time you ask a man how he's feeling and he uses adjectives like "fine," "okay," or "good," it probably means "I don't feel safe enough to be emotionally vulnerable."

Although our strong emotions may or may not be accompanied by tears, it is wise for us to become connected with how we feel and express these emotions to loved ones. Those who develop this ability also report healthier lifestyles and less emotional disturbance.

In working with individuals who have become desensitized and disconnected from their authentic self through perpetual consumption of pornography, it is apparent that many of them need to reconnect with their feelings. One way of doing this is to first become aware of *what* you are feeling. Learning the language of emotion is like learning a foreign language. It requires concentration, focus, and the acquisition of a new vocabulary. You might consider getting a list of feeling words and begin each day to review the list (see Appendix G) and identify words that accurately capture emotions you have had. As you do this, contemplate the circumstances in which your feelings emerge. Be curious about your interpretations of these events and how these interpretations influence your feelings. This process perpetuates a pattern of being more self-aware. You might even consider recording your feelings in a journal and practice sharing them with your spouse. As you become more emotionally honest with yourself and others, you will discover that this behavior creates intimacy between you and your loved ones. You become transparent and others are able to know you more deeply. Your need to feel loved, admired, accepted, and appreciated is met in more profound ways. This is what intimacy is about. Another way of thinking about intimacy is "in-to-me-see." When we are truly intimate with loved ones, we allow them to see inside of us. Transparency is what creates closeness in relationships. Some fear that allowing others to see aspects of their inner selves will place them at risk for rejection. The irony is that by being vulnerable with others, we actually become more real and more attractive and draw others closer to us. Take some emotional risks with your feelings and share them with your spouse. You might be surprised that instead of rejecting you, your spouse may actually feel more attached to you.

As you become more emotionally connected you should begin appreciate the fact that humans can actually experience dichotomous emotions at the same time. For example, we can feel sad and optimistic at the same time. The important thing is to use as many adjectives as you can to accurately identify your internal feelings and then write them down. There is something therapeutic about seeing feelings symbolized in words.

Some time ago, a man listened to his wife express the pain she felt as a result of his choices. Cognitively he understood that he should feel sad and remorseful, but he reluctantly confessed he felt nothing. He was coached through his feelings. "So you feel numb?" He replied affirmatively and was invited to say more. "And what's that like for you?" He replied that it was "frustrating" because he believed he should feel remorse but did not. This was processed further. "So you're feeling confused?" "Yes," he replied. "And disconnected or detached from myself." Interestingly, this man was able, through some small coaxing, to begin expressing his experience with adjectives. He found five adjectives that described his emotions. He said he felt numb, frustrated, confused, disconnected, and detached. Despite his lack of ability to offer his wife empathy for her pain, these five words gave her hope that somehow her husband would be able to engage with her on an emotional level. This gave her a small sense of reassurance that her decision to recommit to the marriage might be profitable after all.

An important side-effect of connecting more authentically with others is that it creates alternative attachments with real people that can eclipse the imaginary relationships developed through pornography use. Although there is the risk of rejection when attempting to connect with real people, the relationships are more meaningful than those you will experience consuming pornography. The actors in pornography will never ultimately satisfy or meet your needs for emotional intimacy.

14. Develop Competing Distractions

We all need to disassociate from problems from time to time. It is important to find some compelling distractions that can compete with the lure of pornography use. Some of our clients have had success developing emergency kits that they use if cravings to act out become so intense that they are difficult to ignore. These kits have included such items as photographs of loved ones, phone numbers of the members of your support network, gift certificates for wholesome activities, inspirational quotes or poems that have personal meaning, letters of encouragement (you can include a letter from yourself or invite your spouse to write a letter of inspiration to help you at times when you're struggling), a list of the consequences of continued pornography use, music, a journal entry, or notecards with helpful concepts gleaned from therapy or conversations with friends and loved ones. It's best to include a variety of items since one item seldom works in every situation. These items can be kept in the car or in a briefcase and taken out at times when you feel like turning to pornography.

In addition to competing distractions, you can work to develop new rituals in your day-to-day routine that break up the patterns that trigger your pornography use. For example, one individual used to act out when his spouse left for a weekly Parent Teacher Association meeting. He developed some new rituals for this night and started attending a community college woodshop class. The new routine disrupted the negative weekly rituals and expectations he had formed. Another person rearranged his office furniture at work so that his computer monitor faced the door and committed to start keeping the office door open at all times. This was a new ritual for him that centered around his patterns related to computer use in the workplace.

15. Be Engaged in a Good Cause

Individuals consume pornography because they feel like it, and they will probably continue to use it unless they feel more compelled to do something else. Many individuals who struggle with pornography say they believe their behavior is selfish. In their recovery, they replaced these tendencies of self-gratification by adopting lifestyles that were less internally focused. A colleague often tells her clients to "get a life." She clarifies this by telling them that they needed to get a life they can feel passionate about and look forward to waking up to every morning. When we're engaged in meaningful endeavors, we find motivation to live more meaningful lives that are less centered on ourselves. Consider opportunities for random acts of kindness or service opportunities.

16. Be Prepared

The time to prepare is today. You need to practice batting the ball long before you're up to bat on the day of the game. Anticipate times where you might be feeling more stressed, anxious, or depressed. Develop strategies that anticipate danger and keep you safe during such moments. Earlier, we gave an example of a man who had his TV removed from his hotel room prior to his arrival. He used the time he would have normally spent viewing pay-per-view pornography to do some journal writing, exercise in the hotel's gym, and write a letter to his wife. He kept himself busy and kept himself safe.

Another individual often acted out when he felt stressed. Having just graduated from law school and preparing to take the bar exam, he decided to check in with his wife daily on how he was doing. This helped deter him from turning to pornography to cope with his stress.

Most individuals know what their vulnerabilities are and the times when they will be most susceptible to indulging in pornography. Being prepared means taking extra precautions, anticipating risk, and preparing strategies that you can turn to during times of high vulnerability.

17. Consider Your Authentic Desires

Desire is more than a passive preference. It is a verb. It is something that we *do!* There are many factors that influence our desires. We should be curious about what determines our desires. What thoughts or behaviors nurture and perpetuate our desires? Do our desires vacillate over time? What makes our desires more or less intense?

The fact of the matter is that until you are able to see the value of self-mastery, self-discipline, and delayed gratification in your life, you probably won't desire these abilities enough to pay the price necessary to acquire them.

Ask yourself what you desire most and check to see if your actions are in allignment with that desire.

One man felt little desire to change because he didn't realize the impact of his choice to compulsively masturbate to pornography. For one thing, his solo-sex activities diminished his desire to pursue his wife sexually. This left her feeling unloved and unwanted. She felt robbed of opportunities to have closeness with him because he developed another relationship with pornography and masturbation. The irony is that this man did desire to be close to his wife but was blind to how his choices were actually creating estrangement in his marriage. He felt victim to the message the adult entertainment wants people to believe: "Indulgence in pornography is harmless fun and it doesn't hurt anyone." The reality of his situation is that it was harming his relationship and hurting his wife. Furthermore, it was hurting him by creating emotional distance in his relationship. As he contemplated what he wanted for his relationship, he realized that his current behavior was incompatible with what he truly desired. This realization began a journey toward recovery. He learned ways to connect with his wife and develop the kind of meaningful relationship that ultimately was more aligned with his authentic desires.

18. Avoid Tunnel Vision

Reject all or nothing thinking. Don't fail to recognize the many markers along the road to recovery. When you lose perspective about recovery because your vision is too narrow, you risk feeling despair and hopelessness about the possibility of change. There is a tendency among those on the path to recovery to measure progress exclusively in terms of their ability or failure to avoid pornographic materials each day. While it is important to monitor target behaviors closely, recovery should be viewed in the broader context of healing and behavior modification. If acting out is the sole basis for monitoring success, you can lure yourself into a false sense of security during times where you are free from acting out, and this can cause you to neglect other important aspects of recovery. Small steps are the most sure. Establish patterns of success by setting flexible, attainable goals and achieving them, even if it means continuing target behaviors while implementing incremental change.

19. Be Creative

It can be tempting to try to pattern your steps to overcoming pornography problems on the successful methods of others around you—particularly if you participate in group therapy. It is a good thing to emulate success, but often the best solutions to your problem lie within you. Don't underestimate your strengths. Have confidence that you can think through your problems and develop creative strategies of your own. Some of the most effective strategies for you will come from you. One client who was in the video production industry recorded himself on video as he spoke about what he really wanted in life. He was careful to say exactly what he knew what he would need to hear when the urge to consume pornography came upon him. He also set up a way for his wife to record a message of encouragement on video each week. These mini-videos were downloaded onto his iPod and when he felt tempted to act out he would just choose one of several videos to watch.

Another man used humor by putting a card on top of his computer monitor at work that read "How's my surfing? Call my wife to report reckless Internet cruising" and it gave his home phone number. This generated a lot of humorous discussion in his office, but later these discussions turned more serious and provided opportunities for several other men at work to approach him and have some genuine conversations about their own problems with pornography use. Together, these men committed to helping keep each other safe at work. This provided an invaluable support network where this man's motivation to change was increased.

Both these individuals decided to be creative and their efforts paid off in meaningful ways. You should be curious about your own ability to come up with unique interventions that are customized to your particular needs and circumstances.

20. Recommitment to Spirituality

For years there has been widespread reluctance on the part of the community of psychologists to embrace spirituality as a therapeutic tool. Issues of spiritual belief have seemed enmeshed with religious dogmas that have been considered repressive. But religion and spirituality are not the same thing. At a base level, we all have some connection to what we would define as spiritual values in our own terms. And the social sciences are starting to evaluate the psychological impact of active spirituality on people's sense of well-being.

Spirituality consists of that which inspires you and moves you towards something transcendent or noble—something greater than yourself. People connect with their spirituality in different ways. For some people, spirituality means congruence between what they see conceptualized as their mind, body, heart, and soul. Others connect with their sense of spirituality through a theological framework such as Christianity, Buddhism, Native American Rituals, Islam, and so forth. Many people also connect with a sense of spirituality through nature, the arts, meditation, relationships, or simply sitting in their backyard and looking into the stars while pontificating about the meaning or purpose of life. Defining what spirituality might mean to you is outside the scope of this book, but we do recognize a pattern among many individuals who successfully abandon pornography that includes a recommitment to spirituality, whatever they personally perceive this to be.

21. Evaluate and Prioritize Your Values and Beliefs

Perpetual consumption of pornography tends to distort and corrupt core values and beliefs about sexuality and people. Many individuals who have consumed pornography for years indicate that they actually begin seeing the men and women around them primarily as objects to be used in their fantasies and sexual gratification. An important aspect of abandoning these perspectives will require you to evaluate and reprioritize your values and beliefs.

You might begin to evaluate your beliefs by writing down your behavior and then retroactively asking yourself what belief might influence such actions. For example, whenever you get a sexual urge or craving do you inevitably act out by masturbating to pornography? If this were true, you might have some of the following beliefs about sexual cravings: 1) sexual feelings are irresistible, 2) sexual cravings will only get worse if I do nothing, 3) sexual urges are more powerful than me, 4) I can't handle my sexual cravings, 5) the only way to deal with these cravings is to act out, or 6) I have to conquer these sexual feelings in order to be free. Beliefs like these are not only erroneous; they render you helpless. Such beliefs are irrational and replacing them with more accurate beliefs can help reduce the amount of intensity that sexual cravings have for you. For example, consider the following alternative beliefs: 1) sexual feelings have a lot of energy, 2) sexual cravings come and go, they will not last indefinitely, 3) these sexual feelings are part of who I am and they're powerful, 4) managing these sexual cravings can be challenging at times, 5) there are several choices I can make about what I will do with these sexual urges, and 6) it will be important to learn to cohabitate and live in harmony with my sexuality.

It would be narrow-minded to limit your evaluations to beliefs only about sexuality. What about your beliefs related to honesty, openness, relationships, marriage, commitment, responsibility, and many other aspects of your life? Once you assess your beliefs you should be curious about whether the beliefs you have written down are really *your* beliefs or someone else's? For example, I believe a particular principle because my spouse expects me to. Has this belief been internalized or merely generated externally?

It is helpful to consider your beliefs from a broad perspective. For example, if someone was considering their beliefs about relationships they might consider what their values are about their relationships with their spouse, with stress, work, pornography, the environment, food, and so forth. What are the characteristics of a healthy marital relationship?

Here are some examples of things people may value in their relationships:

- *Adventure*: to have new and exciting experiences
- *Commitment*: to make enduring, meaningful commitments
- *Courtesy*: to be considerate and polite towards others
- *Dependability*: to be reliable and trustworthy
- *Fitness*: to be physically fit and strong
- *Family*: to have a happy, loving family
- *Genuineness*: to act in a manner that is true to who I am

- *Humor*: to see the humorous side of myself and the world
- *Loved*: to be loved by those close to me
- *Passion*: to have deep feelings about ideas, activities, or people
- *Self-control*: to be disciplined in my own actions
- *Solitude*: to have time and space where I can be apart from others
- *Wealth*: to have plenty of money[2]

Once you have exhausted a list of things people might value, next consider categorizing them into three areas 1) very important to me, 2) important to me, and 3) not important to me. Limit yourself to four or five values that are very important to you. Then, consider whether your behavior reflects these values as being very important. If not, you must resolve the discrepancy between what you profess is most important to you and how you conduct yourself. Ultimately, many people find themselves labeling values as "very important" that are not reflected by their behavior. This is perfectly normal, and in fact, can serve as a template of the type of values you'd like to adopt. For example, you might profess that honesty is very important to you and yet you lie about your pornography problem to your spouse, employer, or others. You should be curious about this discrepancy and how it has come about. This value can represent something you want to work towards. You might say, "Honesty isn't very important to me but I would like to change that about myself. I'd like to adopt honesty as a value that will be very important to me." This reprioritization leads to a set of new values and beliefs that belong to *you*, not someone else.

After you have refined the list of values that you would like to be most important to you, consider what changes you will need to make in order for this to be so. If I chose honesty, I might think about how I would be different if honesty was very important to me and then begin acting accordingly. With this approach, I begin to become the person I want to be.

Summary

This chapter has considered some of the principles that emerge frequently as we work with men and women seeking to abandon habitual pornography problems. These principles can be helpful as you seek to reorganize your life and make incremental progress towards a more healthy view of intimacy and a more meaningful relationship with your spouse. Many of the principles are so much more than just making first-order changes. They involve evaluating several aspects of your life and contemplating what activities or behaviors may influence your minute-to-minute choices. At first, all of the suggestions combined may seem overwhelming and if you try to do them all at once you will find it difficult. Select some of these principles discussed in this chapter as you customize a strategy that might work for you. Share your ideas with your spouse or other loved ones. One of the most effective tools in combating addiction is the support and accountability that spouses bring to each other. Pornography tears marriages apart. But when spouses work together honestly and openly to overcome the problem, they actually strengthen their commitment. Learn to think of your marriage as a tremendous asset to overcoming your problems with pornography together. You might also consider working with a therapist who can provide some objective feedback and help you monitor your change process. As you attempt to implement a strategy for change, take some of these principles for a test drive and see how they work for you. Finally, give yourself training wheels and don't expect to implement them with perfection at first. Change is usually a process, not an event!

Notes

1. Naomi Wolf, "The Beauty Myth" *Harper Perennial,* 2002.
2. Taken from the work of Dr. William Miller and his colleagues at the University of New Mexico

15. Managing Vulnerability after Success

M any people on the path to recovery are frustrated by their inability to maintain behavioral changes over time. Most individuals feel capable of regulating their behavior in the short term but lack confidence about long term sobriety. This chapter will briefly discuss some considerations about managing your vulnerability to pornography over time.

By the time individuals seek help in therapy for pornography problems, they have likely had multiple unsuccessful attempts at abandoning their behaviors on their own. They feel frustrated and exhausted. Many even feel hopeless about the prospects of change. Others, however, seek help with a resolve to change, but the change they envision is dramatic. "I want to get over this once and for all," said one man. Another said "I just want to fix this so it isn't a problem in my life anymore." Such statements reflect how painful their journey has been and also how strong their desires are to be liberated from the unpleasant reality they have created for themselves. In order to really be free however, it is first necessary to understand behavior in context and to gauge realistic expectations. First, we want to briefly revisit the concept of addiction, then talk about sobriety, and finally address ways to maintain gains made during the change process.

The label "pornography addict" is generally applied to those whose lives have been consumed by pornography or who feel compelled to use pornography habitually. Those in favor of applying labels do so in part to break through the minimizing and denial those entrenched in pornography often exhibit to avoid responsibility for their choices. Admitting you have an "addiction" can be a catalyst for seeking help from others. It can be a humbling experience for a person to reach out for assistance and rely on others to provide a road map of how change might occur. People who oppose the label of addiction believe that labels pathologize or stigmatize people because some pornography users will then adopt such labels as self-fulfilling prophecies: "I can't help myself, I'm an addict."

In an attempt to appease both audiences, in this chapter we'd like to categorize those who struggle to abandon pornography as having a "vulnerability." Part of this semantic alteration to the construct of addiction is strategic. People have a hard time accepting they are flawed in some way. This same phenomena explains why people are afraid to get their eyes checked, go for their annual physical examination, and so forth. Instead, consider your problem with pornography a vulnerability. If managed, it's conceivable that you may never act out. However, we'd also like to invite you to consider that because you have created powerful paired associations with pornography, this intoxicating relationship is part of your history and subsequently you will likely always have a vulnerability to pornography if you don't maintain healthy boundaries in your life. If you don't manage this vulnerability, or if you adopt a mentality of "I'm over it" or "I no longer have a problem" after several months of sobriety, such statements in and of themselves might suggest you are at risk of having a relapse.

To further illustrate the concept of managing a vulnerability, consider someone who has been diagnosed with diabetes. They will need to check their blood glucose levels daily and make adjustments with insulin when needed. Additionally, a healthy diet and proper nutrition will be important. This course of action makes diabetes a manageable problem for many so diagnosed. They live very normal lives, and the risks of diabetic shock or diabetic coma remain dormant. What if after two years of managing glucose levels, a diabetic convinced himself that since he hadn't had a problem with glucose levels for two years that he must no longer have diabetes? Similarly, consider the cancer patient who neglects check-ups because their cancer is in remission? In both of these cases, it would be unwise not to monitor the condition or vulnerability. Likewise, those who have developed a pornography habit must be careful to avoid complacency about managing their vulnerability and be mindful of precipitating risk factors throughout their lives if the symptoms of pornography problems are to remain dormant. In order to do this, you might find it more helpful to accept your pornography problem as a vulnerability. This doesn't mean you're flawed and it doesn't mean you're damaged goods. If you're tempted to think this way, let go of these distorted views about your behavior. There isn't a single person, including the authors of this book, that don't possess some vulnerability. It might be a vulnerability to overspending, or a vulnerability to rescuing others from their problems, or vulnerability to mismanaging time, or tendencies to be forgetful, and the list is endless. Your vulnerability is pornography. Accept this and move forward with your life by making the necessary adjustments along the way that will keep you away from harm. When people can be okay with possessing a vulnerability, they seem to feel less anxious about the process of change and do better in maintaining long term sobriety.

Alternatively, there is the other side of the coin. You can try to brush your behavior under the rug, expecting that somehow it will go away. You might like to know that spontaneous remission from these types of problems is rare. Others believe if they haven't acted out for a certain period of time it must no longer be a problem. Neither of these strategies reflects meaningful change. Subsequently, we should take precautions to keep ourselves conscious of those factors that will help us manage vulnerabilities to indulge in pornography. This is especially true in a culture that is so flooded with degrading or fraudulent messages about our sexuality. Keeping safe is about managing the problem. What it is *not* is a plan to extinguish your sexual feelings. Ideally, people are encouraged to learn ways to live in harmony with their sexuality.

The Pitfall of Complacency

When people find themselves returning to old habits, it is usually complacency that takes them back down familiar roads. Because complacency is a precursor to relapse with pornography, strategies to manage complacency should be developed. A lot of men report trying different things to abandon pornography but claim their efforts have failed. Interestingly, while they were actively involved in their treatment plan they report that it worked. They seldom talk about the period of complacency where they lost the momentum to continue doing what was working for them. This issue of complacency is an enormous factor related to people relapsing.

One key to avoiding the trap of complacency is to conceptualize sobriety from a life of pornography as part of a more comprehensive process than simply the presence or absence of your behavior. How will you monitor and track complacency, and what is your plan when you feel yourself getting burned out? How will you rekindle your flame? We don't have the answer to every question, and this is one of those questions that would be important for you to wrestle with a bit.

Maintaining Sobriety

As you seek to maintain sobriety, you might consider how you define sobriety. Most individuals say it's helpful to have a bottom line (e.g. not consuming pornography on the computer). However, you should also have a broader definition that will help you strive towards managing your vulnerability after consumption of pornography has been abandoned.

Our definition of sobriety is: *"Energy, effort,* and *priority* placed on monitoring and managing vulnerabilities and risk factors that precipitate or perpetuate acting out with pornography."

The premise for this definition is that we fall long before we act out, and if we're not actively engaged in efforts devoted to maintaining sobriety then we're at risk for having a relapse.

A steady course of abstinence followed by slips followed by abstinence followed by more slips is not a pattern of healthy change. Change feels different. It looks different. We would expect longer periods of abstinence and, if relapse occurs, we would expect an individual to get back on course quickly. So, when setbacks occur, we get back on our feet and continue pressing forward. Change is possible. It sometimes takes time, but remember that change is about much more than just abandoning behaviors that impair us from developing a more intimate relationship with a spouse.

Studies about relapse prevention have found that one of the most influential factors related to abstinence across a broad domain of addictive behaviors is the level of self-efficacy a person has about change. As noted in the previous chapter, self-efficacy refers to an individual's beliefs about their competence in a particular area. When relapse occurs, it is usually because a person's confidence and perceived control is challenged by a high-risk situation where they begin to doubt or question their ability to maintain sobriety. Research has analyzed episodes of relapse and identified three high-risk circumstances where it is most likely to occur. These situations are 1) uncomfortable emotional states (e.g. feeling depressed or anxious), 2) interpersonal conflict, and 3) social pressure (which might also be conceptualized as societal pressure).[1]

Individuals who are able to develop effective coping responses to high-risk situations reduce relapses significantly. Each experience of coping with urges to act out in high-risk situations increases feelings of self-efficacy and reduces the likelihood of relapse. These moments should be celebrated, as they constitute part of the thousand small moments that cultivate momentum and empower individuals to abandon pornography. The presences of these moments are highly correlated with people's ability to master and manage high-risk situations.

If slips occur, individuals can fall prey to phenomena known as the *abstinence violation effect*. This effect predicts that when an individual has a slip, they will engage in negative self-appraisals about the slip, catastrophize internal dialogue about inabilities to change, experience negative emotions involving guilt or shame, and ultimately feel a reduction in their level of self-efficacy. In many cases where individuals slip, they report being inadequately prepared or being caught off guard in the middle of a high-risk situation.

Successful strategies that appear to effectively help people manage their vulnerabilities usually include 1) developing some coping skills, 2) therapy, and 3) reorganizing lifestyles around sobriety.

Coping Skills

Coping skills vary across different relapse prevention plans. Professor of Psychology at the University of Washington, Dr. G. Alan Marlatt, has studied the process of relapse prevention extensively. He suggests that individuals are benefited by several skills as they manage their vulnerabilities. These include 1) understanding relapse as part of the process of change, 2) learning to identify and cope effectively with high-risk situations, 3) managing cravings and urges, 4) developing a strategy to implement damage control in the event of a slip in order to minimize its negative consequences, 5) continuing treatment, even after a relapse (e.g. continue to attend a support group), and 6) cultivating a more balanced lifestyle.[2] These skills should not be construed as a "nice" list to consider. One of the top peer-reviewed journals in psychology, the *Journal of Consulting and Clinical Psychology*, has published research validating the effectiveness of these skills in relapse prevention.

Therapy

Therapy provides an environment of safety and support. Sometimes it is hard to be objective about your change process, and a separate set of eyes can provide invaluable insight. More importantly, a skilled therapist can ask questions that will help you explore your strategies for change and also identify areas where you may be at risk. Many people feel blind to high-risk situations that catch them off guard and make them susceptible to relapse. A therapist or a support group can see things you may not and help you avoid common pitfalls that lead to relapse. In therapy, you can also be challenged and confronted in an environment where you know people are genuinely seeking your welfare, not trying to demean you or tear you down.

Complacency can also be avoided by continuing to participate in therapy. Those who are working to maintain sobriety become less complacent, especially if involved in a support group. In this context, individuals are encouraged to make sobriety a priority in their life. People are encouraged to take some time every day doing those things that will help keep them safe, similar to the regiment of the diabetic. Many of the things outlined in this book are things that will keep you safe. The following are some things clients report helpful.

1. Be humble enough to accept your vulnerability and responsible enough to have a plan about how you will manage it. Consider how you're

managing things and whether there are aspects of your sobriety that are being neglected. This includes monitoring complacency.

2. Have periodic checkups with a counselor or regularly schedule an appointment to visit a support group or report to a trusted friend on how you're doing. Some clients have an annual or semi-annual checkup with a therapist the same as they do with their dentist or doctor. You should consider monitoring how you're managing stress, revisit some of the concepts that have kept you safe (e.g. identifying and correcting thinking errors), or report on the closest you've come to slipping since your last visit.

3. Evaluate whether you are starting to rationalize or whether you see your problem as the "past." Do you have any hooks that haven't been addressed? One client was asked about his Internet filter during such an evaluation and reported that it had expired. This was rectified and helped him avoid returning to behaviors he had worked hard to abandon.

4. Be motivated about goals you're actively working on. What is the purpose of such goals, and are they congruent with a life of sobriety? As you move through your treatment, these goals will become more focused on healthy lifestyle changes.

5. Reread some of your literature, such as this book, to evaluate how you're doing. Look at worksheets or other materials (e.g. your journal). Reflect on where you're at and what you still want to change about yourself.

6. Ask your spouse to give you feedback on how emotionally connected she feels with you. This is always an important gauge about your process of change.

Cultivate a Balanced Lifestyle

Pornography habits are usually a sign of imbalance in a person's life. The antitheses of chaotic or stressful lives are ones balanced by those things that help you be your best self. Individuals often complain that they have no time amidst the hectic demands of their schedule. We would suggest that if you don't choose sobriety as a priority in your life it will make no difference what you choose instead. Take the time to develop balance! Balanced lifestyles can include a healthy diet, exercise, meditation, time for some type of community service, and recommitment to some type of spiritual practice that helps you connect with your authentic self. These activities contribute to helping you develop and strengthen your coping capacity so the lure of pornography has less energy for you.

Summary

Working through recovery is a process, not an event. People are benefited more if they can adopt a strategy of managing a vulnerability as compared with those who feel the need to "fix" or "extinguish" their problem. Part of managing vulnerability requires monitoring complacency that may emerge as you move further along the road of sobriety. As acting out becomes less of a factor, sobriety should be generalized to assess the *energy*, *effort*, and *priority* placed on monitoring and managing vulnerabilities and risk factors that precipitate or perpetuate acting out with pornography. Strategies to cope in high-risk situations should be developed, including circumstances where you experience 1) uncomfortable emotional states (e.g. feeling depressed or anxious), 2) interpersonal conflict, and 3) and social pressure. Finally, successful strategies that appear to effectively help people manage their vulnerabilities usually include 1) developing some coping skills, 2) therapy, and 3) reorganizing lifestyles around sobriety.

Notes

1. Marlatt, G. A. & Gordon, J.R. (Ed.). (1985). *Relapse Prevention: Maintenance strategies in the treatment of addictive behaviors.* New York: Guilford Press.
2. Parks, George A., and Marlatt, G. Alan (2000). Relapse Prevention Therapy: A Cognitive-Behavioral Approach, *The National Psychologist*, 9(5).

SECTION 4:
Help and Support for the "Other" Spouse

16. What About Me?
Seeking Help and Support

Despite a wife's need for support, when her husband's problem becomes known it is common for the attention of caregivers to be directed toward helping him abandon pornography. Less is offered for the wife. The husband's problem is more clear cut. When it comes to the "other spouse" and their injuries, the terrain changes from a behavioral problems to the strong emotional reactions that naturally emerge when wives feel betrayed by their husband's indulgence in pornography. In some cases, people may feel that if they help the husband they are also helping the wife. But wives who are attempting to support their husband's recovery have real needs too. This chapter is dedicated to helping you, the injured spouse, seek help and support for yourself, not for your husband. It's not about how to "fix" him; it's about how to find reservoirs of strength for *you*. Our experience is that the prognosis for a positive outcome for the relationship is significantly enhanced when wives receive support and help to resolve their pain.

Clarify Roles and Responsibilities

Many women will erroneously blame themselves when they discover their husband's pornography problem. They believe if they were more physically attractive or more sexual, their husbands would not be turning to pornography. This is lie! The majority of these men have a long history of consuming pornography that began prior to meeting their spouse. Wives need to be clear on who is responsible for the pornography problem. We believe a spouse is never responsible for her partner's choice to use pornography! It is also true that a husband's pornography use is not a reflection of a wife's sexuality, attractiveness, or personality traits, but rather a statement about his inability to cope with challenges in healthy ways. Women are not responsible for the problem and are not responsible for fixing it. Wives, your role in a husband's healing process is to seek help for yourself and then support his efforts to abandon his behavior, and, in time, be open to trusting again as positive changes occur.

One reason it is helpful to clarify your responsibilities is that often women own their husband's problem, and as long as she feels obligated to fix it, it is likely her husband will never really assume accountability and responsibility to address his problem. It's interesting how often wives make the phone call to the therapist for the counseling appointments. Women also become the ones who feel responsible to find a computer filter or software program to monitor Internet activities. We've even seen cases where women take full control over managing the budget in order to monitor all financial transactions. You could spend all of this energy seeking support for yourself instead of becoming preoccupied with fixing a problem that isn't yours to fix.

Seeking Support

Wives often report feeling embarrassed or ashamed about their husband's pornography use. This can alienate a wife from reaching out to others. She may fear the consequences of disclosing the problem or fear that people may not understand. Some women have reported feeling afraid that others would judge them. One wife confided in someone she thought was a friend only to be told, "If you were keeping your husband satisfied, he wouldn't be jerking off to porn." Perceptions such as these demonstrate insensitivity and also ignorance about pornography problems. Women should carefully select people in whom they can confide during this emotionally taxing time. Wives might consider family, friends, religious advisors, and professional counselors. Some communities offer support groups for wives of men struggling with various sexual problems. These can be invaluable sources of support.

Another reason to seek support outside the primary relationship is that it is likely a woman will not feel safe turning to her husband when his choices have become the source of her pain. Initially, he may also be devastated that he has been caught or found keeping secrets and, in such states, unavailable emotionally to explore or try to understand his wife's pain.

In some cases men attempt to silence their wives with manipulative pleas such as "If you tell your sister the whole family will know" or "If you confide in our religious advisor I'll never be able to attend another church service." Remember that you are not seeking support for him, you are seeking it for yourself. We might add that if your spouse becomes disturbed or angry at your attempts to seek support from others, you might remind him that he has made *his* choice and has forfeited the right to dictate the consequences of how you will choose to compensate for or react to his behavior.

Care for Yourself

It is essential that wives take care of themselves during difficult times of emotional turbulence. Our society often polarizes the concept of self-care. On one hand, people are told to become self-autonomous, independent, and "connected" with the self to an extreme that can dangerously alienate people from human interpersonal relationships that are often rewarding. The other side of the spectrum occurs when service is rendered to others at the expense and neglect of self-care. We, the authors, advocate a model of caring for oneself that includes balance so fatigue and energy are not depleted to the extent where you lose clarity of mind or you become too impaired to effectively addressing the diverse issues that accompany pornography problems.

As self-care opportunities are explored, you might consider placing a priority on activities that make you feel human, valid, and worthwhile. The following are some examples of self-care activities that women have reported meaningful in their journey of healing:

- Volunteering at a library to read books to children.
- Starting a group where women can meet once a week at each others' homes for a lunch and hiring a chef to teach the group how to cook a new dish of food.

- Learning and applying principles of proper nutrition.
- Joining a health club and starting a regular routine with exercise and proper sleep.
- Learning the art of meditation and finding some time each day to reflect about your life.
- Connecting with a sense of spirituality, however you define it.
- Carefully selecting and reading a self-help book of interest to you.
- Enrolling in a course at a local college or university.
- Going to a spa, getting a pedicure or a massage.
- Learning a new hobby.

This list is intended to get your mind thinking about various possibilities and ways you can cultivate self-care. Part of the purpose of these activities can include opportunities to have a distraction from the temptation to obsess and become preoccupied with thoughts about your husband's pornography problem.

Develop Boundaries

There are many situations where one of the partners in a relationship desperately wants the other to change, but nothing happens. Many women in this situation feel like they only have two choices: put up with it or leave. Wives who feel trapped might consider exploring other alternatives with a trusted friend or a qualified professional counselor. As you receive support and suggestions about how you might establish some boundaries in your relationship, you will discover additional options and choices you may not have otherwise considered. You will likely encounter some turbulence as you try to communicate your expectations. This is common. You may be tempted to perceive your assertiveness as punishment of your spouse and consequently feel guilty. Don't! Such actions are one of the most meaningful ways you can show a spouse you love him. You're saying, in essence, "I care about you too much to stand idly by and let you live beneath yourself." Let your frustration and disappointment about unmet expectations in your relationship translate into a firm love that communicates that behavior unbecoming to your partner is unacceptable in your relationship. If you really want to help him, stop rescuing him from the consequences of his choices.

Establishing healthy boundaries with a spouse involves clarifying limits and implementing structures that help your husband be his best self while protecting yourself from further impropriety and disregard for the marriage. For example, when boundary violations are related to sex, a wife may desire to change the degree of sexual intimacy she is comfortable with so she does not feel used, hurt, or objectified by her husband. He must understand and be sensitive to the fact that when trust has been breeched new ideas of "normal" will need to be negotiated if healing is to occur. Allow yourself time and do not feel obligated to rush this process. It is also important if you decide to redefine your sexual relationship that you do not allow your boundary to be compromised by fear that limits on sex will drive your husband further into his pornography. If he uses your boundary to rationalize and give himself an excuse to consume more pornography, then this provides you with feedback and information that can be used to make future decisions about the relationship. Give yourself a reality check and remember that you do not have the power to *make* your husband use pornography any more than you have the power to *make* him stop. Ultimately, the choice to abandon pornography must be his.

If the primary consumption of pornography has occurred via the Internet, you might evaluate what you would like to see differently about computer usage in the home. If your husband refuses to make changes you will need to consider how you can use this information to decide what you will or won't do. You are not helpless in this situation nor should you feel obligated to become the "porn police."

It is helpful when defining boundaries to 1) identify what is most disturbing to you about his problem, 2) use areas of discomfort to help you decide what your new boundaries will be with him, 3) seek help or support from others as you determine possibilities and options of boundaries to consider, 4) evaluate and explore those things you can control and distinguish them from those you cannot, and 5) focus your energy and effort in those areas where you believe you might have the greatest success in creating positive change in the relationship.

Every woman has a different threshold, and what you need might be very different from someone else in a similar situation. If you feel like you're in crisis mode, slow down, breathe, and do whatever is necessary to help yourself relax enough that you can think creatively about what you will do.

Medication

In some rare cases, and we believe such cases are the exception, some women are so overwhelmed and flooded by the discovery of a pornography problem they deteriorate into a state where they may be a danger to themselves or become so dysfunctional that they feel paralyzed in their ability to complete basic tasks necessary for daily living. In these extreme cases, you might consider discussing medication with your provider as an interim solution until you can regain your capacity to regulate your faculties more effectively. If medications are sought, explore options with your provider to determine if there are solutions that can help take some of the edge off your intense experience that will not blunt or significantly diminish your ability to exercise cognition or creative thinking that will be important as you develop strategies to effectively respond to your challenges.

Become Empowered through Education

Take some time to become educated about pornography problems so you can feel empowered to react to the various issues that may surface as you tackle what probably feels like a daunting task. Becoming educated may occur through books, talking to a counselor, or talking to other women who may have experienced similar challenges. Find books that will educate you about pornography problems. As you become more educated, you will feel empowered to become more objective and see the problem with greater clarity and accuracy. Women will often report a transfer where they feel less of the weight associated with bearing the burden of the pornography problem. This permits them to allow their anger and frustration to become more proportionate to the problem while the behavior itself becomes less personalized internally.

Define Healthy Sexuality

A pornography problem parallels eating disorders in several ways. Specifically in both treatments, there is a need to reorganize the way we think about an aspect of our lives. In an eating disorder, that aspect is food. In a pornography problem, it is sexuality. This is different from substance abuse treatment that often attempts to condition a person to abstinence. It is easy to become focused on all of the dynamics of sexuality that are problematic, but it is harder to draft and develop a definition of what constitutes healthy sexuality. There are a vast array of views about sexuality and what healthy sexuality is and is not. Defining healthy sexuality can be challenging especially with so many mixed messages about sexuality in our society. There are more than 20 professional social science journals devoted to issues of human sexuality that contain a wealth of information to assist people in exploring different models of sexuality. Most universities offer classes in human sexuality. Of course, there is your own subjective experience with sex that will shape and mold your views and perspectives. As you absorb the constellation of values and beliefs about sexuality, you may find it helpful to begin thinking about what will define sexuality for you. What is the purpose of sexual intimacy? What aspects of sexuality am I comfortable with? Why do I value sexual intimacy? How are my views about sexual intimacy similar or different than my spouse's? Does pornography have any place in sexual intimacy? Why or why not? These are among many questions you might ask as you start to develop and define what you would like sexual intimacy to look like in your relationship.

Summary

Although it is common to focus on your husband's behavior, this can be a distraction from devoting energy and effort into seeking your own help and support. There are several things you can do to help yourself, including 1) clarifying roles and responsibilities, 2) seeking support from trusted sources, 3) taking care of yourself, 4) developing health boundaries, 5) considering medication if circumstances are extreme, 6) getting educated and becoming empowered through learning about pornography problems, and 7) beginning to develop your own definition of what you would like healthy sexuality to look like in your relationship. In seeking help for yourself, you indirectly influence your relationship and your husband's choices. As you take time for yourself, you will discover that being in a healthy place will help you develop clarity so difficult decisions and obstacles in the relationship will seem less challenging and you will have the energy and strength to press forward regardless of what your partner chooses to do.

17. Finding Relief, Healing Wounds, and Forgiving

From a mental health viewpoint, physical and emotional fidelity are important traits in stable, satisfying marriages, and while some argue the use of pornography does not violate physical fidelity, it certainly falls into the category of emotional infidelity. When one views pornography in a solitary, secretive manner, they take sexual and emotional energy away from the marriage and into other domains. Consumption of pornography can become a type of competing attachment with the primary relationship. A person turns to pornography to be soothed, escape emotional discomfort, or find stress relief instead of finding comfort and validation with their spouse. Interestingly, many women report that they would have preferred their husbands had had a real-life affair instead of indulging in pornography. One woman reported, "I would actually have retained more respect for my former partner if he had had a relationship with another woman because at least he wouldn't have been seeing women in the ways pornography encourages." Another said, "At least if he would have had a real affair it would have been more demanding for him. A woman would have had expectations for him, emotional needs, a desire to spend time, and he would have had to make some sacrifices and invest some energy. Pornography demanded nothing of him. It was just a cheap thrill and a way to self-indulge and satisfy himself without really having to go out of his way."

As we have noted before, there are often a vast array of issues and concerns a partner has when pornography is discovered. There are a number of factors that impact the degree of concern and initial reaction to a discovery of pornography. For example, the type of pornography (heterosexual, gay, child, transsexual, bestiality, cartoon), the themes (violent, degrading, masochistic, bondage, fetish), the venue in which it was consumed (the Internet, strip clubs, adult entertainment shops, video games) and where it happened (at home, at work, while traveling on business). Usually, most reactions have one particular common denominator: the injured spouse begins to become consumed and obsessively preoccupied with reoccurring thoughts about their partner's use of pornography and what this behavior means to the marriage relationship.

Preoccupation about a Partner's Pornography Use

It's normal to become concerned about the presence of pornography in your marriage. You have a right to understand and know what types of behaviors have occurred. However, caution should be exercised in how much information you seek when asking him about his behavior related to pornography. There are many details about your husband's actions that you have a right to know: How long has he been indulging himself in pornography? When does it happen? Who else knows? What forms of deception has he used to keep secrets from you? Have the children ever been at risk? What are the themes of the pornography he consumes? For example, is it heterosexual? Does it depict violence? If his behavior has escalated to infidelity with others, you have a right to know whether his sexual behavior is putting your health at risk. There is a temptation, however, to want to know details about his fantasies or the content of what he's imagined or seen that is unhealthy. There are aspects about our clients' conduct that we do not want to know. We must be cautious about exploring some aspects of pornographic behavior because we may inadvertently give energy to the things we're trying to avoid.

For some people and in some instances, a spouse becomes preoccupied about the presence of pornography in the relationship and they fixate on this to the point where they find it difficult to focus on anything else. This disturbance is real and can cause emotional distress that impairs your ability to function. Subsequently, we'd like to offer a few suggests about ways you can manage this type of preoccupation. The following are some strategies that people have found helpful.

Normalize: Realize that to some extent, your behavior is common and normal. It's easy to be concerned when we feel that our relationship is being threatened, and this concern can easily translate into excessive preoccupation. You might be interested to know that sometimes *worrying* is a behavior we engage in to avoid the emotion of fear. If we worry hard enough, we distract ourselves from experiencing fear. This too, is a fairly normal human response to a threat.

Reframe: This involves constructing alternative ways to look at this problem that may be less negative. Ask yourself if there is anything positive that might come about because of this discovery? For example, "This will give my spouse and me a chance to become really emotionally honest with each other," or "This discovery confirms my intuition that something was amiss in my marriage, and I'm not crazy for thinking something was wrong."

Construct Alternative Meanings: Develop alternative ways of how you interpret your spouse's behavior. For example, instead of thinking of his pornography use as a reflection of your attractiveness or your ability to satisfy him sexually, conceptualize his behavior as a statement about his inability to cope with stress, emotional pain, or problems in living. One woman reported "I started to feel sad when I realized my husband saw no other way of coping than to turn to his pornographic medication so he could become distracted from his problems." Another said "It made me curious how he was so desperate to feel loved or validated that he would turn to that material even when he knew it was an illusion."

Limitations: Limit your preoccupation to a specific time each day. You may decide to allow yourself 30 minutes a day to think about this problem. Put a timer on 30 minutes, go somewhere you can have peace and quiet, and then obsess intensively for 30 minutes. Write down all of your thoughts, concerns, etc., and dump everything in your head onto a piece of paper. However, when the 30 minutes is up, do not allow yourself to be preoccupied with these thoughts anymore. If you have an urge or desire to start obsessing, just remind yourself you'll have 30 minutes tomorrow to revisit your thoughts.

Distractions: Distractions are a normal part of life. When we go to a movie, we allow ourselves to become entranced and disassociate from reality. These temporary periods of time allow us to avoid the stresses of daily living and relax. You might consider getting a massage, starting a new hobby, or engaging in some random acts of kindness for others. There are lots of healthy distractions that we can pursue that will preoccupy us with alterative things to think about.

Social support: Social support can be an invaluable resource, in part because it is also a distraction. When we're with others, we avoid situations where we are isolated and have time to become preoccupied with the pornography problem.

Be Curious: If you find yourself excessively preoccupied, consider being curious about what *you* gain from habitually focusing on *his* problem. Are you getting distracted from your own issues by focusing on your spouse's problems? Is this drawing energy away from things that would be more productive and efficient uses of your time? Are you using preoccupation as a way of seeking attention for yourself? Do you worry excessively about his behavior as a way of avoiding the painful emotion of fear? What are your worst fears? One woman reported that she had invested 10 years of her life in a relationship and allowed herself to be vulnerable with the man she married, and her worst fear was that she had made a bad choice and that her spouse would never be able to reciprocate the love she felt toward him.

These are a few strategies that can help you contain or manage the tendency to fixate or become preoccupied with your husband's choice to consume pornography. We mention the importance of these approaches to help you cope with the pain you may feel as a result of choices made by your spouse. Additionally, in order to begin the journey of forgiveness, it is often helpful to take care of yourself and make sure you have the energy it will take to begin to be open to the idea of letting go of the pain. If the pain and hurt you feel is so consuming that you are in a chronic state of emotional deregulation, it will be difficult for you to focus on the process of forgiveness.

What Does It Mean to Forgive?

In Chapter 10, we briefly defined forgiveness. We suggested forgiveness is letting go of the right to expect a person to be punished. It means letting go of resentment, maladaptive anger, or hatred towards the other person. Dr. Janis Abrahms Spring, in her book titled *How Can I Forgive You*, deviates from this mainstream conceptualization of forgiveness and suggests what she labels a more "radical" model of forgiveness. Her version of forgiveness requires both the injured party and the offender to collaborate in order for the process to occur. If an offender rejects the invitation for reconciliation, Dr. Spring suggests that forgiveness is not possible, but instead, offers the concept of acceptance to the injured party as a substitution for forgiveness. This acceptance, in part, means grieving the loss of what might have been had the offending partner reciprocated efforts to reconcile. Many people struggle with her model, in part, because it appears at first to contradict morals rooted in Christianity. These tenants of faith suggest forgiveness should be offered regardless of the offenders intentions to make things right.

Letting go of harboring grudges or seeking retaliation against those who have offended us and moving forward with our life, or embracing "acceptance," is consistent with principles that cultivate emotional, mental, and physical well being. This process, however, does not mean that we allow those who have injured us back into our lives, and more importantly into our hearts, without *them* making an effort. If the *other* person doesn't make some sacrifice or investment in the process of healing, the relationship cannot be restored to its former state. If a true process of reconciliation is to take place, it requires two people working together collaboratively to repair and reestablish the relationship. In this sense, Dr. Spring is accurate in saying that forgiveness, or reconciliation, cannot occur without a combined effort of all parties involved in the injury.

Counterfeit Forgiveness

Some women offer forgiveness too quickly without requiring something from the party who has injured them. How is forgiveness offered when your husband has no idea about the impact of his choices in your life? What specifically are you forgiving him for? In many cases, you might be offering him counterfeit forgiveness because you're trying to keep the peace. You sacrifice any validation of your hurt and pain to avoid ruffling feathers. You might even see yourself as being responsible for his choices and so you "owe" him a pardon. In some instances, you might even join him in his rationalizations, such as "He's under a lot of stress." In the end, what you're offering him is superficial. It's a counterfeit and ultimately it will not be appreciated or have any value. It will buy you nothing in the long run. Counterfeit forgiveness leads to the same dead end as counterfeit money—the relationship will be bankrupt and have no value, and you'll feel imprisoned by your choice to avoid holding your husband accountable. What he really wants is for you to communicate that his behavior is unacceptable and that you love him enough that you will not stand idly by and let him live beneath himself. In most cases, counterfeit forgiveness is a way of silently consenting to his behavior, which will usually continue or get worse.

Withholding Forgiveness

The opposite extreme of counterfeit forgiveness is withholding forgiveness. You allow his actions to fester inside you until you become completely consumed and preoccupied with what has happened. You maintain your victim role and continue to hold regular pity parties long after people have stopped coming. You reject any attempts by the offending party to reconcile. You believe no one understands how deeply you've been hurt, when, ironically, *you* have yet to wrestle the complete truth and depth of your own emotional pain. People with more severe cases of withholding forgiveness often seek opportunities to punish and avenge the wrong or injustice you've experienced. Suggestions for ways to resolve the injuries are pessimistically appraised and then rejected. You rationalize your position by chronically revisiting the deficits in the other person's attempts to adequately address your grievances while simultaneously offering them no specific road map to guide their efforts. Slowly you begin to alienate yourself from loved ones and friends who feel drained in your presence, as you perpetually recount old events or share the latest episode in a series of never-ending stories that portray how unfair life is to you. Many people who withhold forgiveness see every subsequent catastrophe in their life as a consequence of their partner's original mistakes, and they become blind to their own accountability for the person they have become.

Clarity about the Injury

Regardless of the ultimate outcome of how your spouse chooses to respond to your invitation to reconcile the relationship, it is an important part of healing to develop some clarity about what has been painful for you. What is it about the nature and extent of the damage that hurts so much? Are there secondary wounds? (e.g. Are you equally disturbed by the deception as you are about his pornography habit?) How has this behavior affected you? Of everything that has been painful, what hurts most? What do you expect or hope your partner will do? How can you help him understand your needs? Can you evaluate your husband's choices independently of his behavior? How can you establish boundaries that will prevent further hurt? What are you currently doing to facilitate or prevent any reconciliation process? What markers will provide evidence that your partner is willing to address the injury? What signs might suggest your husband is not willing to pay the price necessary for reconciliation, and what will you do if these signs become evident?

Identifying Your Own Needs

In order to express and invite your husband to address the injuries that have occurred, we want to share with you common processes we see among many couples who successfully confront and overcome pornography problems in their marriage. This process takes time. It is not a quick fix. But sometimes slowing things down allows us to see things we might have otherwise overlooked. The process of resolving pornography problems usually involves the following items:

1. The partner who has consumed pornography develops the ability to regulate and process their own feelings *and* respond to their partner's emotional needs.

2. Distorted beliefs about the self and about one's spouse are transformed to healthy adaptive beliefs. For example, "I'll never have my needs met in this relationship" might transition to "If my partner understands *how* to meet my needs, I believe my partner will try to meet them."

3. A road map for restoring trust is established that clearly outlines what would be necessary for the injured spouse to begin trusting again (e.g. regular disclosures, placing a filter on the Internet, emotionally honesty, etc.).

4. The injured partner feels that the other partner understands the impact of his choices to consume pornography and they become sensitive to addressing ways to resolve the injury.

5. Both partners in the relationship have some experiential evidence that their decision to recommit to the relationship will not be regretted.

6. Objective insight, awareness, and understanding of each partner's unhealthy choices occur.

7. Both partners begin to reorganize their feelings and beliefs about their sexual relationship around new realities.

8. New patterns and rituals for accessing, connecting, and responding to each other's emotional and physical needs are established.

This list is not intended to be comprehensive. Each couple will negotiate and collaborate on their own terms to heal their relationship. These patterns also come with a price tag. Perhaps the first thing to be said of attempts to heal wounds is that things can get worse before they get better. It's like a visit to the doctor's office when you are hoping for pain relief and he instead inserts a needle of stinging lidocaine into the heart of your wound. The pain can be a little shocking. This is natural and to be expected. In time, however, if both partners truly desire to reconcile their differences, real progress can be made.

What If My Partner Doesn't Respond?

If a partner does not appear to desire reconciliation, step back from the situation and try to evaluate it objectively. Sometimes the discovery of a pornography problem can be so devastating that it skews the way we see things. For example, you may have restructured some of your beliefs about the relationship or your partner (e.g. he doesn't want to be with me or he doesn't love me anymore). This can translate into what psychologists call *attention bias,* where your attention is biased by your new belief. This influences the way you interpret your experiences, and you begin to look for evidence to support your new belief and often filter or ignore evidence that contradicts your perception. For example, is it possible that your husband does desire to reconcile but is afraid, ashamed, or humiliated. He may believe he is a failure and that the prospect of resolving the problem is hopeless. Some husband's engage in what has been labeled *strategic self-limitation,* where they fear taking any further risks they believe may result in further loss, suffering, or regret. Others simply do not know how to respond. They're emotionally cut-off or disconnected and don't know where to begin.

If you look at things objectively and still feel like your spouse is non-responsive, it is helpful to revisit your own needs and find what it would take for you to be willing to remain in a relationship plagued by habitual pornography consumption. How will you use this information to make choices about the future of the relationship? Are there ways you can encourage your spouse to reconsider or take some risks? If they still do not respond, how will you communicate your feelings about their choice?

One woman told her husband she was going to leave him for 60 days and give him time to think about their marriage and what was important to him. But instead of considering possibilities for reconciliation, he binged on pornography the entire duration of the separation and began patronizing strip clubs where he paid for sex. His wife was healthy enough not to blame herself for his choices but used this information instead to make a decision about the marriage—she divorced him. Interestingly, she did not dissolve her marriage in anger or hostility but with sadness that her partner was unwilling to resolve their differences. She later reported that to stay in the marriage and allow him to continue his behavior would have only further diminished his self-worth and self-respect. She saw the divorce as an act of benevolence both for herself and her husband.

Transfer of Responsibility for the Injury

Other situations have had different outcomes. Husbands have responded and recognized the importance of addressing the grievances of their spouse. Many had no idea how offensive or hurtful their behavior was. These individuals sincerely desired to reconcile and change their behavior. One interesting aspect among other couples where the wife sets limits and boundaries was a transfer of responsibility for the problem. The wife became less concerned because the husband began being accountable and responsive to her needs. This is a very common occurrence among couples who work through pornography problems in a healthy way, and it is a sign that change is occurring.

When the offending spouse is serious about making things right, they are often unsure where to begin or what they must do. Over the years, we've invited these individuals to write down some questions that would indicate their willingness to explore how their choice to consume pornography has impacted their partner. The following questions are examples taken from individuals who really desired to repair the damage caused to the relationship but knew they must first explore the extent of pain their spouse experienced as a result of their behavior. These questions demonstrate an effort to be a "witness" to the pain and suffering of their spouse. In these discussions, husbands learned to validate and empathically respond to the impact of their choices. Their wife's response to these questions harvested information that empowered these men to offer a more *accurate*, *specific*, and *genuine* apology:

- What has it been like for you to have the sacred trust you placed in me betrayed through my choices?
- How do you experience your days differently now than before the discovery of my behavior?
- What ongoing events or activities trigger painful feelings for you? How often do these experiences occur?
- How have my choices impacted your beliefs and feelings about intimacy in our relationship?
- What boundaries would you like to establish, renew, or change about our intimacy?

- What fears do you currently have about me or our relationship? When are these fears more intense? What helps reduce your fear? How do you physically experience fear (e.g. bodily sensations, headaches, tension, restlessness etc.)?

- What aspects of our relationship need to be reorganized or redefined in order for you to feel more safe? What boundaries are you currently uncomfortable with?

- What things need to change in order for you to feel like you could begin to be open to start trusting again?

- What aspects of my pornography consumption are most offensive to you?

- What aspects of this problem am I closed about? How do I shut you down from expressing your feelings? What is one thing I can do differently to help improve our discussions about difficult topics?

- To what extent do you feel trapped because of my decisions? How can I help you feel like you have more options and choices?

- What impact have my choices had on spirituality in our home or in our relationship?

- As I work towards restoring trust in our relationship, what are some specific things I will need to pay attention to? What things can I change that would give you some hope?

- How can I check in with you on a regular basis to let you know how I'm doing? What things would you like me to report or disclose to you?

- Would you like me to get some counseling? Would you consider joining me for couple's therapy so we can explore options with someone who might be able to help?

- What do you see as being the most important priority for our relationship at this time?

- In all that has happened, what has been the most painful aspect of your experience?

- What do you need most right now in our relationship?

In group therapy, individuals who take responsibility for their choices act very differently than those who do not. One man felt he didn't need to disclose or check-in with his wife because this felt like he was in "kindergarten." Besides, he claimed "why should I check-in with my wife when things are going well because it will just stir things up again." A more mature member of the group offered to let this man view a page in his therapeutic journal titled "Why I Should Check-In With My Wife Even When Things Are Going Well." Below this he had written the following:

1. This is probably on my wife's mind, even if I'm not thinking about it.

2. Regular disclosure will help my wife be more supportive of my goals.

3. I want my wife to have all the information she needs so she can make informed decisions about our relationship.

4. Regular disclosures will help me avoid the secrecy that often perpetuates these problems.

5. Regular disclosures, including days when I struggle, will help my recovery seem more realistic to her.

6. Checking-in will help me establish a pattern of honesty in my relationship.

7. If I don't report regularly, her imagination about what I'm not telling her will probably be worse than anything I will disclose.

8. Reporting to my wife about my progress will demonstrate an effort on my part to be sensitive to any residual anxiety she may have about this problem.

9. I have breeched the trust in my relationship and this is something I can do to help restore trust that I have violated.

10. Regular disclosures can help me avoid complacency or apathy that can precede a relapse.

This is an example of how men who have consumed pornography have taken responsibility for their choices. They own the problem and their wives are able to slowly let go of worrying about it.

Authentic Forgiveness

Authentic forgiveness is one of those phenomenon that occurs while couples are being vulnerable with each other, making sacrifices for the relationship, and taking risks to repair damage caused by injuries each has experienced. At some point during this process, people are able to let go of the pain, the anger, the frustration of unmet expectations, and see the injury with greater clarity and objectivity. They remember the injury because the scar is still there, but somehow, the power of the wound to hurt as it once did subsides and healing occurs. When this phenomenon occurs, people don't ask us, "How will I know when I've forgiven him?" They just know in their heart that some transformation has taken place. Despite what initially seems like a one-way injury with a clear offender and an easily identifiable victim, couples who experience authentic forgiveness often report that each of them find themselves offering a genuine apology and explicitly communicating to the other, "I forgive you."

There is confidence that as a couple they can tackle challenges in their marriage and find success. Both partners recognize that the relationship isn't immune to future injury. Naturally, in the course of life, intimacy requires risk-taking, and risks are always accompanied by the possibility of setbacks and challenges. Dedication and commitment to a meaningful relationship can be antidotes to threats that would undermine the union. As couples restore trust, mutual acceptance, and reciprocation of affection, each is nurtured and nourished by the relationship. They eventually arrive at a healthy place where they can grow and cultivate a loving companionship, the one they always envisioned the day when wedding vows were made.

New Normals

As couples work through the process of reconciliation (or in some cases couples may choose to dissolve the relationship, especially in cases where a spouse shows no effort towards change and is habitually consuming pornography), new normals will be developed for the relationship. Seldom do people want things to really "go back to normal." Despite the undesirable consequences of pornography problems, many couples report that issues which surfaced as a result of pornography forced both partners to develop more effective communication skills, abilities in validating and being empathic towards each other, and problem-solving strategies in the midst of conflict and emotionally charged situations. These abilities, though hard won, ultimately benefit most couples.

As couples work toward establishing new normals, the greater context should be a development of healthy attachment that will empower each individual to thrive and grow. Healthy attachment evolves in relationships as partners become accessible and responsive to each other and share the intimacies of their lives together. Consistent accessibility and responsiveness to various needs in the relationship creates the safety, security, and context for emotional vulnerability and mutual engagement to occur. In order for these new normals to emerge, each partner has to focus on the other person, accurately understand each other's needs, and respond to those needs in a manner consistent with traits that cultivate intimacy. In this greater context, many couples report satisfying and meaningful relations.

Summary and Conclusion

It's hard to summarize what we feel is in itself a brief summary and overview of the many hours we have spent with couples where one partner has become entrenched habitually with pornography. We have tried to offer a glimpse into the lives of men and women whose relationships have been impacted negatively by pornography. Despite our best efforts, we are confident that we have probably raised more questions than we've answered. Yet we hope we have illuminated the constellation of issues that can surface when marriages are threatened by the impact of compulsive pornography use. Even more, we have desired to provide some clarity and direction that will give couples hope that their marriage can survive pornography problems. Is this always the case? No. Statistically some marriages are dissolved, but usually in such cases, pornography was not the only factor that impacted the relationship. Most couples genuinely desire closeness that comes from cultivating healthy intimacy.

We hope that the information contained in this work will augment that process for you and your spouse.

APPENDICES

A: Is Pornography Addiction Real?

Some people wonder whether it is possible to become addicted to pornography. The answer to this question depends on how the word *addiction* is defined. Addiction is often associated with powerlessness, illness, or disease. These words may portray the individual as having little control over his behavior. Many mental health professionals reject this model of addiction, maintaining that it runs contrary to counseling's assumption that people have the ability to control their behavior and change their actions. Perceiving addiction as an illness or disease also runs the risk of having the client justify his behavior. For example, a client may think, "I can't help myself because I'm an addict." Thus, the behavior may inadvertently be reinforced through such categorizations. Furthermore, the DSM-IV (Diagnostic and Statistical Manual of Mental Disorders), used by mental health professionals to diagnose clients, does not contain an entry for "pornography addiction."

Many outside the mental health profession also remain skeptical about the connotations of addiction as applied to compulsive pornography use. In the wake of some dramatic accounts about addiction, a *Newsweek* headline mocked, "Breathing Is Also Addictive."[1]

One definition of *addiction* reads, "devotion: a great interest in something to which a lot of time is devoted." Another suggests being addicted is "to devote or surrender (oneself) to something habitually or obsessively."[2] Both these definitions suggest that addicts actually choose their habitual, destructive use of pornography. Therefore, it is also their choice to get help in stopping such behavior. Clinical experience has shown that abandoning heavy pornography use is at best extremely difficult if not impossible without outside support and intervention. Individuals must, however, earnestly choose to receive this help in order for it to be successful.

Although the debate about pornography as an addiction continues, the mental health profession is faced with determining how to diagnose and treat people whose lives are being adversely affected by their habitual use of pornography.

One argument suggests that behavior associated with pornography consumption should be categorized as an obsessive-compulsive disorder (OCD) instead of an addiction or impulse control disorder. The most important distinction between these two definitions lies in the fact that addicts *escape* discomfort while those who suffer from OCD *avoid* perceived negative experiences. Dr. H. J. Shaffer defines the difference as follows:

> The loss of insight among addicts and the maintenance of discrimination among OCD sufferers distinguishes these populations. While the excessive behavior patterns of OCD are disconnected from the dysphoric affect that energizes their activity, addictive behavior remains attached to these noxious emotions. Consequently, addicts *escape* their discomfort by acting out through excess behavior patterns, while OCD patients *avoid* the conscious experience of psychic pain through repetitive intemperate activity.[3]

Dr. Jennifer Schneider argues an alternative view that symptoms related to habitual use of pornography align more closely to the diagnostic criteria for substance dependence disorders.[4] An examination of the similarities presents some interesting findings. Keep in mind, only three of the seven criteria need be met in order for someone to be clinically diagnosed with a substance dependence disorder (an addiction). The following items are taken from the DSM-IV. References to *substance* in these criteria generally refer to drugs or alcohol but we have added additional commentary indicating how someone involved with pornography could fit each criteria:

1. The person acquires tolerance, requiring "increased amounts of the substance to achieve intoxication or desired effect." This is a common element among many clients who are aroused by a few images of pornography initially but later spend hours surfing hundreds of images to achieve or sustain their arousal.

2. "Withdrawal symptoms are evident." Many clients report being irritable when they are not able to use pornography. One client became very upset when his wife cancelled a night out with some friends and wanted to spend the evening with him. He had purchased a new web cam and was looking forward to participating in cybersex that night on his computer while she was away with her friends.

3. The "substance is often taken in larger amounts or over a longer period than was intended." It is not uncommon to have clients report spending more time than intended on the computer in pursuit of pornography and viewing more images than they initially intended. Many clients report they were first simply curious but this behavior eventually led to exorbitant amounts of time being consumed by their "curiosity."

4. "There is a persistent desire or unsuccessful efforts to cut down or control substance use." Most individuals seek help after their own efforts to stop using pornography have failed.

5. "A great deal of time is spent in activities necessary to obtain the substance, use the substance, or recover from its effects." The emphasis here on the amount of time being spent to obtain, use, or recover from use corresponds to the thrill some pornography users report from the pursuit to find the "perfect" image or picture—more than from the sexual gratification itself once they have found it. They get a rush from the challenge.

6. "Important social, occupational, or recreational activities are given up or reduced because of the substance use." Many pornography users report greater social detachment, abandonment, and isolation due to increased consumption. Isolation actually fuels interest in pornography

and creates an environment where it thrives. Thus, one treatment goal is to have clients structure environments and schedules that are relatively free of solitude.

7. "The substance use is continued despite knowledge of having a persistent or recurrent physical or psychological problem that is likely to have been caused or exacerbated by the substance." An individual might continue using pornography despite suffering depression, sleeplessness, poor work or school performance, anxiety, etc. He may engage in sexual behavior that places his health at risk. In some cases, individuals have put their lives in danger by meeting strangers offline whom they've met in chat rooms.

One argument against classifying compulsive use of pornography in the same category as substance related disorders is the lack of evidence that, like drugs or alcohol, there is such a thing as physical dependence on pornography. Dr. Patrick Carnes addresses this issue by suggesting that habitual consumption of pornography creates a mood-altering experience that makes the addict feel normal. Without it the addict feels inadequate. This is a pathological relationship with, and dependency on, the sexual experience. Many addicts are so driven by the need for this "fix" that they describe it as physical.[5] An extension of this concept has led several mental health professionals to work with scientists to explore the reactions in the neurochemistry of the brain during pornography use. If the reactions prove to be sufficiently adverse, pornography could be labeled as harmful to the body under the medical model.

Another possible explanation for some type of physical dependency on pornography appears when an individual masturbates while using sexual imagery. During masturbation a link is forged between the pornography and the temporary euphoric feelings caused by the chemicals released during orgasm. Consequently, a dependency is created upon the entire experience in order to attain the desired sexual "high." Similarly, a cocaine addict isn't addicted to cocaine as much as he is addicted to the dopamine released by the brain when he uses cocaine. Pornography triggers fantasies that perpetuate a chain of events ultimately resulting in euphoric feelings. This may be why many producers of adult material encourage masturbation. Engaging in such behaviors powerfully reinforces the continued use of pornography to trigger the subsequent mood-altering experience.

Dr. Harvey B. Milkman and Dr. Stanley Sunderwirth, in their book *Craving for Ecstasy*, discuss neurobiochemical responses in the brain during sexual self-gratification. They discuss arousal, satiation, and fantasy. Arousal is often associated with the neurotransmitters norepinephrine and dopamine, satiation with gamma-aminobutyric acid and endorphins, and fantasy with serotonin.[6] Dr. Schneider states, "It is important to observe that sex can easily fit into any or all of the foregoing categories, making it an extremely powerful mood-altering activity."[7] Although a person doesn't get addicted to pornography, they appear to get hooked on the mood-altering experience facilitated and triggered by the use of pornography.

Nonetheless it is important to observe that just as everyone who drinks does not become an alcoholic, people who use pornography are not necessarily addicted. In fact, the late Dr. Al Cooper found that less than 8% of individuals who engaged in online cybersex and pornography considered themselves addicted, according to several criteria outlined in the largest on-line survey ever conducted on this subject. Dr. Cooper reported that this 8% spent more than 11 hours per week online and suffered varying types of adverse effects as a result of their behavior.[8] He further identified users in three categories: (1) recreational users, (2) sexual compulsive users, and (3) at-risk users (meaning there was a high risk that such users *could* become compulsively active with pornography and cybersex). Dr. Cooper offers an explanation for the onslaught of demands for illicit adult material through the Internet. He identifies three components that make this avenue attractive for someone who may already be prone to sexually compulsive behaviors: the *accessibility*, *affordability*, and *anonymity* provided by the Internet. The three A's provide an opportunity to satisfy curiosity without a high risk of being discovered. Many who would not spend money at a strip club or risk traveling to a bookstore where they might be recognized have fallen prey to the accessibility, affordability, and anonymity of pornography use on the Internet.[9]

Unfortunately, too many of these same individuals get caught in the trap of pornography addition.

Regardless of one's conclusion regarding the addictive nature of pornography, those who are struggling or have loved ones struggling with habitual pornography use fully understand the very real effects of such behaviors.

Notes

1. Steven Levy, "Breathing Is Also Addictive," *Newsweek*, December 30, 1996/ January 6, 1997, 52-53.

2. *Merriam Webster's Collegiate Dictionary,* Tenth Edition

3. Shaffer, H.J. Considering two models of excessive sexual behaviors Addiction and obsessive-compulsive disorder. Sexual Addiction and Compulsivity 1 6-18, 1994.

4. Jennifer Schneider, M.D., Ph.D., practices internal medicine and addiction medicine in Tucson, Arizona.

5. Dr. Patrick Carnes is a well known psychologist who lectures and writes extensively on the topic of sexual addiction.

6. Milkman, H., Sunderwirth, S.: *Craving for Ecstasy.* Lexington, M.A., Lexington Books, 1987.

7. Schneider, J. Addictive Sexual Disorders. *Norman Miller Principles & Practice of Addictions in Psychiatry,* 1997.

8. *Sexual Addiction & Compulsivity* Vol. 7 (1-2) 2000, 7.

9. Cooper, A. (1998). Sexuality and the Internet: Surfing into the new millennium. *CyberPsychology & Behavior,* 1(2), 181-187.

B: Choosing a Therapist

Many people find it difficult to abandon behaviors related to pornography problems without a professional counselor. Below are several suggestions to help you choose a therapist.

1. Does the therapist have state licensure? Is he or she in good standing? Has anyone ever filed a complaint?

2. What are his or her credentials and educational background? How long has he or she been practicing (note that studies about length of experience do not necessarily correlate with an individual's ability to do effective treatment)? Does he or she have any special training in the area of pornography and sexual addictions? How many clients has he or she treated with issues similar to yours? Ask for some referrals.

3. Is the therapist currently accepting new clients? What are his or her hours of availability? Evenings, weekends? What does he or she charge for an initial consultation? Regular sessions? Cancellation fees? How long are sessions? Does he or she offer a sliding scale to accommodate various income levels? Does he or she bill third party insurance companies?

4. How far is his or her office from you? Where is the office located? A clinic, hospital, or private agency?

5. What theoretical perspectives does he or she use? Psychodynamic, behavioral, cognitive, humanistic, existential, experiential, transpersonal? (Ask the therapist to explain the difference in these modalities so you can understand how they will be interacting with you in treatment.) Does he or she facilitate or offer any group therapy for pornography-related

behaviors?

6. When speaking to the therapist, did you feel like he or she was genuinely interested in you? Did he or she take time to answer your questions? Do you believe he or she understood you? Is this someone you feel you could open up to and share your confidential issues with? Do you believe he or she possesses values and beliefs consistent with your goals? Does he or she seem like the type of individual who will explore various options with you and help you recognize areas for improvement? Do you feel like you can trust him or her?

The therapeutic relationship you establish with your counselor will have a significant impact on your success. Take the time to investigate and find the therapist you believe will best meet your needs.

C: Assessing a Problem: Pornography Questionnaire

There are various stages in the road to developing a compulsive habit with pornography. Some individuals may move through these stages in a matter of months or even weeks. For others, it may take years.

Dr. Kimberly Young and Dr. Victor Cline, both specializing in addiction therapy, have created slightly different variations of these stages in their respective publications.[1] Understanding these stages can help you determine how a severe problem may have developed. Note that these stages are not always sequential. Furthermore, it is possible that an individual can experience some of the stages and not others. For example, a person may go through the first three stages, fixate on a certain type of pornography, and remain there for an extended period of time. To assume that the person will move automatically to the next stage may result in an inaccurate assessment of the problem.

1. *Discovery.* The thrill or arousal associated with the material is encountered during this stage. This can happen accidentally or through curiosity. This stage usually refers to initial exposure rather than exposure over a prolonged period of time. There can be a rush because the event represents entering an area that is taboo, forbidden, or simply sensually arousing.

2. *Experimentation/Exploration.* This stage is characterized by various cognitive distortions as the person rationalizes exploring or experimenting with the material: "It's just harmless fun" or "This isn't hurting anyone." Masturbation usually accompanies this stage, powerfully reinforcing the experience.

3. *Desensitization.* As exploration and experimentation continue, desensitization takes place. In this stage, what was once shocking or

atrocious is now considered normal or even mundane, thus setting the stage for escalation.

4. *Escalation.* During this stage, the material becomes rougher, kinkier, or more bizarre in order for the person to achieve the same level of arousal or rush.

5. *Performance.* Frequent exposure to the material introduces many sexual behaviors which a person may want to act out. This stage is characterized by a person mimicking behavior he has seen depicted in the pornography. In some cases, he may attempt to experiment and act out these behaviors with his spouse, or he may seek a partner outside the marriage.

There are a number of questions that can help determine which stages a person has experienced. The pornography questionnaire below can gather a great deal of information about the extent of a problem. The following items provide an outline for questions a therapist might ask a client who presents him or her with a pornography problem. It may not be important for a spouse to know the answers to some of these questions, and in fact, a therapist may not ask all of them. These questions may be repeated throughout treatment because a client may not disclose some answers early on in therapy.

Pornography Questionnaire

1. When were you first exposed to pornography? How old were you at the time?
2. Were you by yourself or with someone else? Whom were you with?
3. What were the circumstances surrounding this exposure?
4. When is the first time you masturbated to pornography? What were your feelings afterwards?
5. How and where have you been accessing pornography? Work, home, school? Other places?
6. Who else knows about this? Why seek help now?
7. On average, how often and how long is each incident?
8. Have you spent more time than you anticipated in pursuit of pornography?
9. Have there been any extended periods of abstinence? When and for

how long?

10. How many times have you unsuccessfully attempted to abandon pornography use?

11. Has the type of pornography gotten rougher, harder, or more bizarre or kinky over time?

12. Have you consumed illegal pornography? Illegal is defined as (a) Ultimate sexual acts, normal or perverted, actual or simulated; (b) Masturbation, excretory functions, and lewd exhibition of the genitals; and/or (c) Sadism and masochism

13. Have you viewed any pornography depicting bestiality, homosexuals, sadism, masochism, bondage, dominance, children, or transvestites? Has any other fetish been eroticized?

14. Have you ever paid money for pornography? How much and where did the money come from?

15. Do you have subscriptions or memberships to porn material? How many? Via email, web sites? How much have you spent for these?

16. Do you print out images on paper or store them on a phone or PDA to take with you during the day?

17. Have you ever met anyone offline that you met online? What happened? How often?

18. Do you have sexualized conversations via chat rooms, newsgroups, web cams, CU-See-Me technology?

19. Do you have pornography sites bookmarked or added to your browser favorites?

20. Do you manually delete cookies, temporary Internet files, and browser history? Why?

21. Do you have any sexualized usernames or nicknames online? How many?

22. Have you masturbated with a partner while online? By yourself?

23. Do you try to hide your online behavior from others? Whom? Have you ever been caught?

24. How often are you online after midnight? All night?

25. Do you feel anxious, angry, or disappointed not being online?
26. Do you ever ask your spouse to perform acts depicted in porn? What is your spouse's reaction?
27. Do you visualize pornography to facilitate arousal during sexual relations with your spouse?
28. Do you store images on your hard drive for later recall? How many?
29. Does your employment require Internet access? Do you have other reasons to be online?
30. Has your consumption interfered with other aspects of life? How?
31. What are your feelings about therapy?
32. How has your spouse reacted?
33. What do you want to do about this behavior?
34. How will we know that treatment has been successful? What will it look like?
35. Is there anything I'm not asking that I should be asking in order to understand this problem?
36. Would you be willing to take a polygraph test to help validate the information you've provided in this assessment?

Although these questions are intrusive, they are not intended to humiliate or shame an individual, nor are they considered all-inclusive. They provide insight for someone struggling with a pornography problem and also help assess and determine how severe a problem may be. Once this is accomplished, appropriate counseling and resources can be enlisted to address the problem.

Notes

1.   Cline, B. Victor, PhD. *Pornography's Effects on Adults and Children*. New York: Morality in Media, 2001; Young, Kimberly, PhD. *Tangled in the Web*.

D: Common Thinking Errors

Unhealthy thoughts produce unhealthy behaviors. A common denominator among individuals with pornography problems is the erroneous thinking they entertain in order to indulge in their behaviors. One of the original authors on thinking errors is Dr. Stanton E. Samenow. The following list of thinking errors has been derived from his work.

1. *Minimizing.* This thinking error involves attempting to make behavior appear insignificant or unimportant. Minimizing is used to avoid responsibility. Minimizing often involves vagueness, being unclear or non-specific, so the listener doesn't have a complete picture of all the details and may be led to draw inaccurate conclusions about the behavior. Examples of minimizing include statements like "I just looked at pornography a few times" or "it's not that big a deal."

2. *Entitlement.* The idea of entitlement means you believe you deserve special treatment, consideration, privileges, or rules because you are unique or special. When your expectations are unmet, you may become agitated, annoyed, or angry. Part of entitlement may involve unrealistic expectations on the fallacy that things should be fair. If someone else gets something, you should too. Feelings of entitlement may also result when people have a grandiose view of themselves. Examples of entitlement include statements like "I've been under a lot of stress lately and this is my way of coping" or "This is just something guys do."

3. *Assuming.* You make assumptions when you believe you know what others feel, think, or are doing without verifying the facts, and then guiding

your actions by these beliefs as if they were true. This thinking error is often used to draw incorrect conclusions that help justify your own behavior. Examples of assuming include statements like "I didn't think you'd care" or "I figured you knew I was doing this since other guys do."

4. *Redefining.* This error involves shifting the focus off an issue in order to sidestep responsibility, accountability, or to avoid suffering consequences. This redefining attempts to avoid solving the problem at hand. It may include answering a different question, one you want to answer and not the question asked. It can often include vagueness or manipulation. An example might include a statement like "I might use pornography but it's no worse than all the soap operas you watch." The intent with this statement might be to shift the focus to the wife's behavior and avoid a discussion about the pornography use.

5. *Rationalizing.* The self-talk or thoughts entertained in order to give yourself permission to act according to your desires characterizes rationalizing. This often involves logical arguments we construct in order to justify behavior and convince ourselves that it's okay. Rationalizing is a thinking error generally used *before* you act. A common application of rationalizing is reflected in statements like "It's not hurting anyone" or "It's not a real-life affair."

6. *Justifying.* Justification involves giving explanations and reasons for your actions in an effort to make the behavior seem okay. Justifying recognizes the behavior but attempts to reject any belief that the behavior was wrong. Justifying is a thinking error generally used *after* you act.

7. *Generalizing.* This thinking error involves taking evidence from a small sample and applying it globally to everything. Generalizations often include words like *never, always, every,* and *only.* Individuals prone to generalizing think in terms of absolutes or extremes. In this same category we find black and white thinking, sometimes referred to as polarizing or the "all-or-nothing" perspective. For example, events or people are sometimes viewed as all good or all bad. Individuals who struggle with pornography problems have difficulty seeing themselves as good people who are making bad choices. They tend to see themselves as bad, shameful, or evil.

8. *Compartmentalizing.* Compartmentalizing involves inconsistencies in professed beliefs and behaviors. It may involve fluctuations in the way you behave in front of people within short periods of time. Individuals often convince themselves they are being consistent when they are not. Some believe they can act inconsistently in various aspects of their lives without having the behavior affect the way they act in all areas of their lives. In order to compartmentalize, you will disown or split parts of yourself. For example, you might embrace your religious beliefs to the point of being rigid and inflexible while disowning your sexuality. On the other hand, you might mentally reject your religious beliefs in order to embrace your pornography use. The antithesis of compartmentalizing is to be an integrated person in your beliefs, values, thoughts, feelings, and behaviors.

9. *Catastrophizing.* This error involves believing that a small problem is so much worse than it really is. It may involve magnifying details about a situation as though the entire ordeal will create a disaster or horrifying event. This often includes black and white thinking. When you catastrophize things, you lack perspective and adopt a tunnel vision mentality. For example, one man got into a fight with his wife. This fight and the negative emotions associated with it were catastrophized to the extent that he began to believe that the marriage was unsalvageable and doomed to be a failure. This subsequently led him to feeling hopeless and then pornography and masturbation were used to escape his emotional discomfort.

10. *Personalizing.* Personalizing involves believing that you are the cause of some negative external event, for which you are not primarily responsible. It also involves thinking that everything people do or say is some kind of reaction to you. For example, one man had his work critiqued by several colleagues. He was deeply hurt by their comments as he had spent a great deal of time on the project. He personalized this by translating their critiques into a belief that he was flawed, imperfect, and less than adequate.

11. *Victimstance/Self-Pity.* This is the position you take when you are held accountable for your actions. You believe that you are not responsible for your actions and that you are the victim. This thinking error often includes

blaming something or someone else for your behavior. It can also involve making excuses to explain, avoid, or justify. Victimstancing can include the belief that things should be fair. Examples of this thinking error include statements like "You never give me sex" or "I've had a hard day at work." Your life may be challenging and you may have difficulties, however, everyone can make a case for being a victim of something and this doesn't justify using pornography. If you require empathy or understanding when you're feeling down, there are healthier ways of having your needs met.

12. *Lying.* This thinking error is a power play. Lying is used to confuse others, to distort information, to avoid taking responsibility, and to embarrass or humiliate others. You use lying to create turmoil and confusion so those around you can never be sure what is going on. Lying serves three different purposes. First, it can be used to make you look good. Second, lying can be used to avoid responsibility and consequences. Finally, lying is sometimes used to intentionally hurt others. Types of lying may include (a) *Commission*—making things up that are not true. Denial and being ingratiating can be part of this (b) *Omission*—Giving some information that is true but leaving out important parts of the truth. Being vague could be an example of lying by omission. Selective memory is often a tactic used to avoid accountability as the person claims he does not remember something when in fact he does (similar to "playing dumb"). (c) *Assent*—Allowing others to believe you agree with them when you do not. Pretending to go along with other people's ideas when you really have no plan to, or agreeing with them just to look good in their eyes, when in fact you have no intention of going along with this or do not really agree.

13. *Manipulation.* Manipulation involves attempts to control by arranging, influencing, tampering, managing, or maneuvering situations or people in a way that you take advantage of or exploit someone or something to get personal gain. Manipulative behavior is often considered devious or shrewd. Ingratiation is a form of manipulation which attempts to find favor with someone for the purpose of getting something from them in return. It is laden with expectations and has a hidden price tag—"I'll be nice to my spouse so I can get sexual favors." Lying can also be a form of manipulative

behavior. Becoming emotional, such as demonstrating anger to get your own way, is a tactic that is considered manipulative. Power and control, religiosity, victimstancing, being phony, and drama and excitement can also be forms of manipulative behavior.

14. *Power and Control.* This thinking error involves using power plays whenever you don't get your own way. You feel uncomfortable when you're not in control, so you use power plays either physically or psychologically on other persons to try to take control. You believe that you have the right to control others, including the way they think or act, but that they do not have the right to control you or make any demands of you. You enjoy fighting or arguing for the purpose of being right or having power—the issue may be secondary. You get a charge or high from overcoming and dominating others. You find enjoyment when others submit to your wishes and desires. Issues related to this thinking error are manipulative and can include many of the forms of manipulative behavior as you try to acquire power and control.

15. *Closed-Channel/Avoidance.* Closed-channel thinking is being secretive, closed minded, self-righteous, and not open to information about yourself from others. It is not being open to new ideas and avoiding any effort at self-criticism or self-awareness. Closed-channel, avoidant thinking is used to divert issues and to conceal the truth. It can be a form of lying, specifically involving lying to yourself. It attempts to maintain some power and control over others by keeping part of your life a secret. This form of distorted thinking is used to maintain the belief that no one is smarter than you and that you can't be wrong, regardless of the situation. The lack of receptivity to feedback and isolated secret thoughts tend to delay personal growth and progress. More dangerous, however, is that this type of thinking tends to continue to fuel and enable inappropriate and unhealthy behaviors that hurt not only you but also those around you.

16. *Pride.* This distorted view of self and others is rigid and inflexible. You refuse to compromise, often on insignificant things. You want to feel good and always be right. Pride is the perception that you are better than others, even when this is clearly not the case. This thinking error is manifest by grandi-

ose views of yourself, a sense of entitlement because you are somehow unique, special, or different from everyone else. Prideful people often feel a sense of ownership over others and are condescending in their mannerisms toward them. Prideful people often present a good-guy image by building themselves up with a few good details about themselves while eliminating or minimizing the negative. Pride is often viewed as self-centeredness, conceit, boastfulness, arrogance, or haughtiness. Prideful people seek to be authorities to themselves and do not like to be subordinate or submissive to the rules of others or of society at large, especially if the rules stand in their way of getting what they want. C.S. Lewis noted "Pride gets no pleasure out of having something, only out of having more of it than the next man. . . . It is the comparison that makes you proud: the pleasure of being above the rest."[1] Pride is contentious, self-seeking and self-gratifying. Pride often prevents people from being humble or submissive enough to be open to change and feedback from others. As a result, prideful people live in their own distorted perception of reality and continue to engage in inappropriate or unhealthy behaviors.

17. *Objectification.* This type of thinking views other people as objects, void of any human qualities such as feelings or thoughts. The person objectifying perceives the object as something that exists for his pleasure. This type of thinking leads a person to fixate on the aspects of another person's body while fantasizing.

In identifying thinking errors it is important to note that they are not mutually exclusive. It is possible to integrate several thinking errors in one statement. For example, after being confronted by his wife for using pornography, one man said "I've been under a lot of stress lately and you haven't been very understanding." He used *entitlement* to suggest that the standard of fidelity in the marriage didn't apply to him because of his stress. He used *redefining* by shifting the focus of attention to his stress rather than his inappropriate behavior. He engaged in *justifying* as a way of making his behavior appear less serious since he was having a difficult time. Prior to acting out, it is evident he used *rationalizing.* He told himself it was okay to use pornography since he was under a lot of stress and his wife wasn't been understanding or sensitive to his challenges. He perceived himself as a *victim* of his wife's lack understanding. In part, he was *blaming* her for his poor choice to use pornography to cope with his problems. He likely used *assuming* by interpreting his wife's behavior as a lack of understanding. Just because he thought his wife didn't care doesn't mean he was right. He never gave her the chance to say she cared and correct his distorted thoughts. The fact that he was caught by his wife suggest he engaged in *lying* to keep his behavior hidden from her. As this example illustrates, one statement can integrate many thinking errors and this is often the case when an individual is defending his pornography use.

Notes

1. C. S. Lewis, *Mere Christianity*. New York: Macmillan, 1960, 95.

E: Maladaptive Toxic Shame

D r. Patrick Carnes, one of the pioneers in assessment and treatment of sexual addictions, suggests two core beliefs that sex addicts have which relate to their fundamental view of themselves. These beliefs are (1) I am basically a bad, unworthy person and (2) No one would love me as I am. Much of the literature addressing pornography and sexual addiction refers to this type of self loathing as unhealthy, maladaptive, or toxic shame.

Many theorists and researchers believe that toxic shame is a powerful driving force in the lives of those struggling with inappropriate, compulsive sexual behaviors. One author, who has written extensively on the role toxic shame plays in addictive behaviors, helps us differentiate between healthy shame (or guilt) and unhealthy "toxic shame." He states, "healthy shame is the emotional core of our conscience. It is emotion which results from behaving in a manner contrary to our beliefs or values." It is the awareness and feelings that say, "I have done something wrong," which then results in a healthy sense of guilt. Toxic shame conversely says, "I have done a bad thing, therefore I *am* bad, I *am* flawed, I *am* defective." He indicates that this form of shame "is the root and fuel of all compulsive addictive behaviors. It fuels the addiction, then regenerates itself."[1] Figure 1 ("Shame Cycle") shows how this regeneration occurs.

Individuals who are shame driven often engage in behavior which some describe as a "double life." While appearing to live a normal, even exemplary lifestyle, they simultaneously live in a world of compulsive, sexual acting out, cloaked behind a veil of secrecy. Some have called it a "Dr. Jekyll and Mr. Hyde" type of existence. These people have learned to cope with the pain of their shame by self-medicating and escaping to a world of addiction or compulsive behaviors. Patrick Carnes says of these individuals, "Sex becomes confused with comforting and nurturing. Therefore, to feel secure means to be sexual."[2] These behaviors generate even more shame in the individuals because of the internal incongruence created by behavior being contradictory to their values and the principles acquired in their family, culture, or religious community. People compensate for this shame by moving to the "control phase" as illustrated in Figure 1. This phase features certain personality traits and behaviors which indicate a need for control or an appearance of stability, or both. These traits may include rigidity, self-righteousness, blaming, pleasing, placating, fanaticism and being critical of themselves or others.

Many addicts become increasingly excessive in the demonstration of these behaviors in their attempt to hide from or compensate for their sense of shame. This becomes exhausting and unmanageable. One individual, in describing his control phase, stated, "I thought if I just worked harder or did everything everyone wanted me to do, I wouldn't feel so bad for what I had done. But I found myself feeling like an elastic band getting wound tighter and tighter. I became more irritable and critical of my wife, kids, and people at work. It finally felt like it was too much to handle. My elastic finally broke and I fell back to my sexual medication to feel some relief and escape, only to start the whole cycle all over again."

The current thinking in the treatment of sexual addictions is that even if there are long periods of sobriety, unless the shame issues are addressed and resolved, the individual will return again and again to the undesired behavior.

A thorough treatment program (1) helps the individual learn strategies and tools to help stop the compulsive behavior, and 2) addresses and heals the toxic shame issues thus changing his unhealthy core beliefs. The exhaustive motion of the shame cycle is brought to a halt and the individual then may return to a healthy, fulfilling life.

Shame Cycle

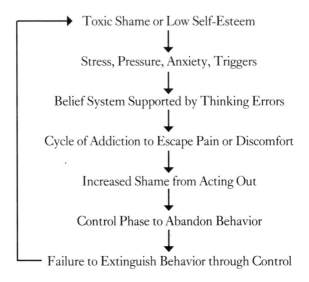

Toxic Shame or Low Self-Esteem

↓

Stress, Pressure, Anxiety, Triggers

↓

Belief System Supported by Thinking Errors

↓

Cycle of Addiction to Escape Pain or Discomfort

↓

Increased Shame from Acting Out

↓

Control Phase to Abandon Behavior

↓

Failure to Extinguish Behavior through Control

FIGURE 1

Control Phase

Compulsive (Excessive) Behaviors: May include working, cleaning, eating, spending, and helping others.

Personality Traits: May include rigidity, self-righteousness, blaming, pleasing, placating, fanaticism, and being critical of oneself or others.

Notes

1. Bradshaw, J. *Healing the Shame that Binds You*. Health Communications, Florida 1988, 15-16.
2. Carnes, Patrick, PhD. *Out of the Shadows*. Hazelden Press, Minnesota 1992, 77-81.

F: Severe Sexual Behaviors Promoted by Pornography

Pornography promotes a wide variety of behaviors. Some individuals move beyond softcore pornography to pornography that is considered bizarre, illegal, or against the norms of normal sexual conduct. This could include pornography involving children or depicting paraphilias, bestiality, or other behaviors for which a person may face legal action.

If you have developed any of the following behaviors in addition to your pornography use, or if you find yourself attracted to pornography depicting these behaviors, it is imperative that you seek professional counseling immediately. Since these are unfamiliar to many, they are described briefly below as taken from the DSM-IV.[2]

Exhibitionism: Sexual arousal derived from exposing one's genitals to a stranger.

Fetishism: Sexual arousal to nonliving objects such as clothing articles. Clients with a fetish usually masturbate while in possession of the object. In some cases they may ask their partner to wear the object during their sexual relations.

Frotteurism: This involves touching or rubbing against a partner who is non-consenting. This behavior usually occurs in a crowed place such as a shopping mall, a train or bus station, or a busy downtown street.

Pedophilia: Involves sexual attraction or activity with a prepubescent child (usually age 13 or younger.)

Sexual Masochism: Involves sexual arousal derived from being humiliated such as being beaten, raped, bound, handcuffed, or subjected to some other form of suffering.

Sexual Sadism: A partner to sexual masochism, sadism involves sexual excitement from the psychological or physical suffering, including humiliation, of others. Someone involved in sadism often seeks a partner who suffers from sexual masochism to act out their fantasies. This is often referred to as S&M pornography or dominance and bondage.

Transvestic Fetishism: This is sexual arousal from a man wearing women's clothing (cross-dressing).

Voyeurism: A person with this paraphilia, nicknamed a "peeping Tom," observes unsuspecting persons, usually strangers, who are naked, in the process of undressing, or engaging in sexual relations.

In the case where disclosure does involve paraphilias, obtain and consult with a professional counselor who has experienced working with these issues. Although disclosure of paraphilias can be difficult, many partners are also willing to work on these issues with their spouses.

Notes

1. The DSM-IV is the Diagnostic and Statistical Manual of Mental Disorders published by the American Psychiatric Association. This is the manual used by mental health professionals to diagnose mental health disorders.

G: Adjectives to Express and Describe Feelings

Pleasant Feelings

Open: Reliable, easy, amazed, free, interested, satisfied, receptive, sympathetic, accepting, kind, understanding, confident.

Happy: Delighted, overjoyed, ecstatic, gleeful, thankful, festive, satisfied, glad, cheerful, sunny, great, joyous, lucky, fortunate, merry, important, elated, jubilant.

Alive: Thrilled, liberated, provocative, impulsive, playful, courageous, free, frisky, animated, optimistic, spirited, wonderful, energetic.

Good: Encouraged, clever, surprised, content, peaceful, at ease, quiet, certain, relaxed, serene, free, easy, bright, comfortable, blessed, calm, reassured, pleased.

Love: Admired, affectionate, devoted, attracted, loving, passionate, warm, touched, sympathetic, close, considerate, loved, sensitive, tender, comforted.

Interested: Intrigued, inquisitive, affected, nosy, snoopy, engrossed, curious, concerned, absorbed, fascinated.

Positive: Confident, hopeful, anxious, inspired, determined, excited, bold, brave, daring, challenged, optimistic, reinforced, enthusiastic, eager, keen, earnest, intent.

Strong: Certain, unique, dynamic, tenacious, hardy, impulsive, rebellious, secure, haughty, overbearing, free, sure.

Difficult or Unpleasant Feelings

Angry: Hateful, indignant, unpleasant, frustrated, annoyed, upset, boiling, hostile, offended, infuriated, bitter, aggressive, insulted, resentful, inflamed, provoked, irritated, enraged, cross, sore, mad, fuming.

Depressed: Detestable, despicable, abominable, diminished, despairing, sulky, bad, abandoned, lonely, dissatisfied, lousy, miserable, repugnant, discouraged, guilty, disappointed, disgusted, ashamed, terrible, powerless.

Confused: Doubtful, indecisive, embarrassed, shy, tense, uneasy, stupefied, skeptical, distrustful, misgiving, upset, disillusioned, perplexed, uncertain, unbelieving, pessimistic, hesitant, lost, unsure.

Helpless: Inferior, useless, frustrated, paralyzed, fatigued, empty, despairing, distressed, woeful, forced, pathetic, tragic, incapable, alone, vulnerable, dominated, hesitant, submissive.

Indifferent: Bored, dull, nonchalant, neutral, weary, preoccupied, cold, disinterested, lifeless, insensitive, reserved.

Afraid: Worried, frightened, threatened, cowardly, intimidated, anxious, terrified, timid, wary, shaky, suspicious, alarmed, nervous, scared, uncomfortable, restless, doubtful, panicked, fearful, quaking, menaced.

Hurt: Rejected, afflicted, aching, victimized, abandoned, devastated, offended, tortured, crushed, heartbroken, agonized, appalled, humiliated, wronged, alienated, injured, tormented, pained, dejected, deprived.

Sad: Tearful, sorrowful, pained, grieved, anguishing, desolate, desperate, pessimistic, unhappy, lonely, mournful, dismayed.